SURVIVE

Disclaimer

This book details my personal experiences with and opinions about survival, and herbal first aid. The statements made about the products and services have not been evaluated by the U.S. Food and Drug Administration. They are not intended to diagnose, treat, cure, or prevent any condition or disease. Please consult with your own physician or healthcare specialist regarding the suggestions and recommendations made in this book.

Except as specifically stated in this book, neither the author or publisher, nor any authors, contributors, or other representatives will be liable for damages arising out of or in connection with the use of this book. This is a comprehensive limitation of liability that applies to all damages of any kind, including (without limitation) compensatory; direct, indirect, or consequential damages; loss of data, income, or profit; loss of or damage to property and claims of third parties. This book provides content related to physical and/or mental health issues. As such, use of this book implies your acceptance of this disclaimer.

Although the publisher and the author have made every effort to ensure that the information in this book was correct at press time and while this publication is designed to provide accurate information in regard to the subject matter covered, the publisher and the author assume no responsibility for errors, inaccuracies, omissions, or any other inconsistencies herein and hereby disclaim any liability to any party for any loss, damage, or disruption caused by errors or omissions, whether such errors or omissions result from negligence, accident, or any other cause.

Dedication

I dedicate this work to my husband Jwan, and my four heartbeats Journey, Jamai, Justice, and Jeremiah. Thank you for keeping me forever inspired.

Preface

Survive is not just a book about what to do if you get stuck in the wild. This topic is based on a combination of over 15 years experience researching and using herbs, as well as an education background in social work. This book combines the knowledge of herbal medicine, wilderness survival, urban survival and human behavior all wrapped up into one. What I have learned over the years in my experience is that people do not have the sufficient tools they need to handle most if not all of life's challenges. Let's face it, we might not ever be in a situation where we are stuck in the wild. However, we might end up in a situation of job loss or severe depression. Survive is a book written to give you not only the tools necessary to survive in life but also if you are in nature.

I used a wide variety of sources and resources to create this book. I used medical manuals, mental health journals, and a host of textbooks to give the reader a vast variety of knowledge. This book may feel like multiple books in one. The goal was to provide one book that has everything you need to know about survival in a simple and easy to understand fashion. There are skills that we need to have in order to survive. This book touches not only on first aid, herbal first aid, and basic wilderness skills, but also how to survive in the concrete jungle.

This book is organized over seven chapters. Chapter one is titled The Human Body. No herbal book is complete without discussing the human body. No herbal remedy nor first aid measure is effective without first having knowledge of the human body and all its functions. The human body is a beautiful and intelligent design, capable of the most amazing feats. This includes healing itself.

Chapter two (Basic First Aid) and three (Herbal First Aid) talk about First Aid. In each chapter you will see common situations where herbal and basic first aid is required as well as herbal remedies that you can use to address them. This chapter also outlines the best methods to administer the herbal remedies to maximize their effectiveness.

Chapter four is called Situational First Aid. This unique chapter outlines common situations that we face outside of the human body that can cause crises. For example, job loss and food shortages. This chapter includes tips to help get you through these tough situations.

Chapter five is Mental/Emotional First Aid. It outlines one of the most underrated conversations around mental health. Mental health issues are on the rise and it is apparent that people are struggling with managing the issues of life. This chapter outlines common mental health issues such as anxiety and anger. It also provides both practical and herbal means of addressing these issues.

Chapter six (Survival Skills) and seven (Survival Kit) both address basic survival skills and how to put together your own survival kit. These chapters also discuss a list of what survival skills you need to know in order to survive both in the wild and concrete jungles.

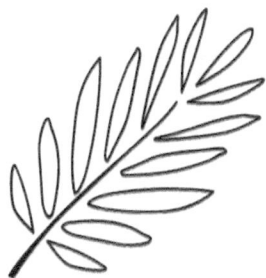

TABLE OF
CONTENTS

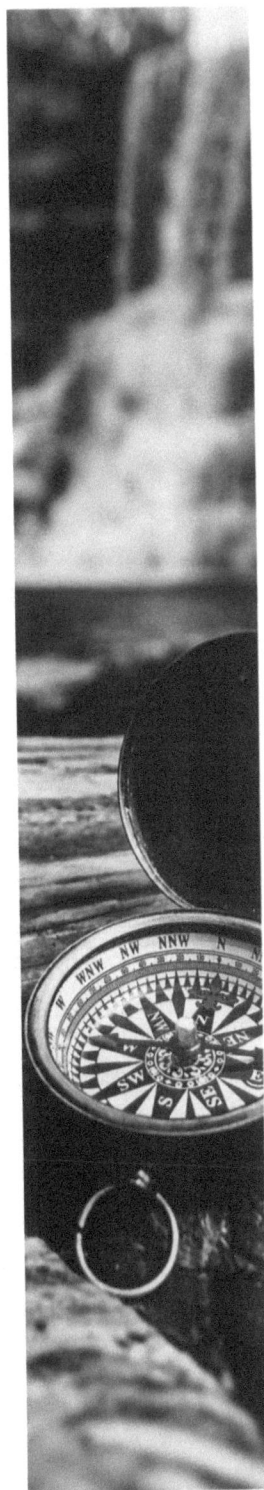

Sur·vive

/sər'vīv/
Continue to live or exist, especially in spite of danger or
hardship.

These are uncertain times that we are living in. Food shortages, inflation, unclean water and food, illness, poverty, homelessness, job loss, fires, and mental health issues are on the rise. My question to you is,

"What are you going to do?"

What are you going to do if the medications that you relied on are no longer available? What are you going to do if the electricity goes out for longer than a few days? What are you going to do if the grocery stores shut down and no more food becomes available? What are you going to do when the doctors tell you that they have done all they can do, just go home, and get your affairs in order? What are you going to do if you are stuck in the wild and need a way to protect yourself? What are you going to do when you are fired from your job or you go through a terrible divorce? What are you going to do when you are overwhelmed with grief of the loss of a loved one? Are you prepared? The preppers of yesteryear are not sounding so crazy now are they? No matter what your philosophy, preparation is always in order. You never know what situation you may find yourself in that could change the course of your life. It could be as simple as a scrape or as severe as a heart attack. No matter what the situation, it is best to be prepared.

Do you have the mental and physical fortitude that is necessary to survive?

I created this comprehensive survival guide in an attempt to provide information on how to handle almost every emergency situation that you might find yourself in. I've included many herbal remedies to help you prepare your own herbal survival kit. Herbs have been used for thousands of years to address many situations that arose during those times. These remedies were effective and that is why many people all over the world are turning back to our ancient medicine.

THE HUMAN BODY

It is important to understand the body's systems in order to correctly formulate remedies and preform first aid. All remedies must work to support the body's own processes to heal itself.

- Integumentary System (skin, hair, subcutaneous tissue)

- Skeletal System (bones, cartilage, ligaments, bone marrow)

- Muscular System (muscle, ligaments, tendons)

- Nervous System (brain, spinal cord, nerves, eyes, ears)

- Endocrine System (pituitary gland, parathyroid gland, thyroid gland, adrenal gland, thymus, pancreas, gonads)

- Cardiovascular System (heart, blood, blood vessels)

- Lymphatic System (spleen, lymph nodes, thymus, lymphatic vessels)

- Respiratory System (lungs, trachea, larynx, nasal cavities, pharynx)

- Digestive System (stomach, intestinal tract, liver, pancreas, esophagus, salivary glands)

- Urinary System (kidneys, urinary bladder, urethra)

- Reproductive System (ovaries, uterus, mammary glands, testes, prostate gland, external genitalia.

- Excretory System (skin, liver, large intestine, lungs, kidneys)

In this section we will look at all the systems of the human body as well as the organs that make up these systems.

Section Key

Organs: This section lists the organs of the system.

In Balance: What the system looks like when it's working efficiently.

Out of Balance: What the system looks like when there is dis-ease in the body.

Organ Affinity: List of herbs that are drawn to this organ system.

System Actions: Actions the herbs need to have on this system.

INTEGUMENTARY SYSTEM

The skin regulates the body's temperature. It protects us from UV light, water loss and microorganism entry. It also has sensory receptors that allow us to feel hot, cold, pain, touch, or other various sensations. This system is the site for melanin production which is a skin pigment protein that protects the hair, skin, and nail color. Melanin is produced in cells called melanocytes.

Organs of the Integumentary System

Skin- Protects the body from fluid loss and microorganisms.

Hair- Organs of sensation and skin protection.

Glands- Secrete sweat and sebum (natural oils).

Nails- Protective plates in the fingers and toes.

In proper balance:

The skin can efficiently produce vitamin D, excrete wastes, protect us from microorganisms, properly regulate our body's temperature, and give us the ability to detect various sensations such as hot, cold, and pain.

Out of balance:

Issues such as bacterial or fungal infections, rashes, dry itching or flaking skin, inflammation, hair loss, or acne.

Organ Affinity

Calendula (Calendula officinalis)
Chamomile (Matricaria recutita)
Chickweed (Stellaria media)
Coleus (Plectranthus scutellar.)
Evening Primrose (Oenothera L.)
Licorice (Glycyrrhiza glabra)
Neem (Azadirachta indica)
Witch Hazel (Hamamelis)

System Actions

Antiseptics
Anti-inflammatories
Astringents
Disenfectants
Emollients
Rubefacients
Styptics
Vulneraries

SKELETAL SYSTEM

The skeletal system supports the structure of the human body, makes blood cells, stores minerals and protects organs. A thin membrane called periosteum covers the bones. The periosteum (a fibrous sheath that covers bones) has two shapes, flat (i.e., plates of the skull) and tubular (i.e., long bones or femurs). There are about 213 bones in the human body.

Organs of the Skeletal System

Muscles- Provides movement, support, and protection.

Cartilage- Provides cushion at the joint's surfaces.

Tendons- Attaches muscle to bones.

Ligaments- Attaches bone to bone.

In proper balance:

When the skeletal system is in balance, bones are strong, organs are protected, and they produce enough red blood cells.

Out of balance:

The osteoblast (bone formation) and osteoclast (bone resorption), processes are hindered. Causes Pagets's disease, bone tumors, osteolysis, osteoporosis, low bone density, bone cancer, and infections.

Organ Affinity

Blue Cohosh (Caulophyllum thalic.)
Blue Vervain (Verbena hastata)
Bonset (Eupatorium perfoliatum)
Horse Chestnut (Aesculus hippo.)
Horsetail (Equisetum arvense)
Juniper Berry (Juniperus communis)
Poke Root (Phytolacca decandra)

System Actions

Analgesics
Anti-inflammatories
Antispasmodics

MUSCULAR SYSTEM

The muscular system is composed of muscle fibers that control the body's movement. There are three types of muscles, smooth (lines the blood vessels, organs and stomach), cardiac (lines the heart and pumps blood around the body), and skeletal (attached to bones and can be consciously controlled). There are over 600 muscles in the human body.

Organs of the Muscular System

Skeletal Muscle- Helps the body move.

Smooth Muscle- Rids body of toxins and helps with digestion and nutrient absorption.

Cardiac Muscles- Pumps blood throughout the body via the heart.

In proper balance:

Heart muscles are involuntarily contracting so that the heart can pump blood efficiently, food is properly digested, and skeletal muscles are strong.

Out of balance:

Muscles weakness, fatigue, muscular wasting, heart issues, inflammation of the muscles, difficulty breathing, and myoglobin leakage (a condition that leaks a protein called myoglobin into the bloodstream and is directly toxic to kidney cells).

Organ Affinity

Barberry root (Berberis vulgaris L..)
Cascara Sagrada (Frangula pursh.)
Lungwort (Pulmonaria spp)
Meadow Sweet (Filipendula ulmaria)
Poke Root (Phytolacca americana)
Stone Root (Collinsonia canadensis)
White Willow (Salix alba)

System Actions

Analgesics
Anti-inflammatory
Antispasmodics
Antiviral
Antiparasitic
Immune Stimulating

NERVOUS SYSTEM

The nervous system uses electrical and chemical means to allow the parts of the body to communicate with each other by relaying messages to various parts of the body. The brain uses chemicals to transmit information and the nervous system uses electrical signals.

Organs of the Nervous System

Brain- Controls all the functions of the body including our thoughts and emotions etc.

Spinal Cord- Relay's messages (sensory, autonomic, and motor) from the brain to the rest of the body.

Sensory Organs- Collects information from the body's sensory receptors and monitors the body's internal and external conditions.

Nerves- Body's electrical wiring that transmits signals from the brain and throughout the rest of your body.

In proper balance:

They communicate proper signals to ensure proper functioning of the body's parts, such as breathing, sexual development, regular heartbeat, movement, and digestion.

Out of balance:

Nerve injury can prevent messages from being sent to certain parts of the body and thus could cause degeneration of nerve cells, blood flow disorders, tumors, autoimmune disorders, numbness, pins and needles feeling, pain, crushed nerves, and neuropathy.

Organ Affinity

American Ginseng (Panax quinq.)
Blue Vervain (Verbena hastata (L.)
Bungleweed (Ajuga reptans)
California Poppy (Eschscholzia calif.)
Cramp Bark (Viburnum opulus)
Passion Flower (Passiflora)
Prickly Ash (Salix alba)
Saw Palmetto (Serenoa repens)

System Actions

Antispasmodics
Nervines
Parasympathetic Stimulants
Relaxants
Stimulants
Soporifics
Sympathetic Stimulants

ENDOCRINE SYSTEM

A network of glands and organs that regulate and control different functions of the body, such as growth, how our organs work, and metabolism. They do this by creating and releasing chemical messengers called hormones.

Organs of the Endocrine System

Hypothalamus- Controls your hormone system.

Pituitary- The "Master" gland that controls the functions of the other endocrine glands.

Thyroid- Regulates the growth, metabolism, and development.

Parathyroid-Regulates calcium in the blood.

Adrenals- Produces hormones that regulate stress, metabolism, immune system, and blood pressure.

Pineal Gland- Creates melatonin and links communication between the nervous system and the endocrine system.

Ovaries- Produces eggs for reproduction and reproductive hormones.

Testes- Creates sperm and the hormone testosterone.

Pancreas- Contains enzymes that help you digest food and helps regulate blood sugar.

In proper balance:

Proper control of growth, mood and development, control of body/water balance, and regulate calcium blood levels.

Out of balance:

The body's ability to regulate processes in the body are hindered causing hypothyroidism, diabetes, adrenal insufficiency, and overactive thyroid.

Organ Affinity

Astragalus (Astragalus membrana.)
Ashwagandha (Withania somnifera)
Chasteberry (Vitex agnus-castus)
Holy Basil (Ocimum tenuiflorum)
Lemon Balm (Melissa officinalis)
Licorice (Glycyrrhiza glabra)
Milk Thistle (Silybum marianum)
Oak Straw (Avena sativa)

System Actions

Adaptogenic
Estrogenics
Tonic

CARDIOVASCULAR SYSTEM

The cardiovascular system, sometimes called blood-vascular system, comprises of the heart, arteries, veins and capillaries. The cardiovascular system delivers oxygen, nutrients, hormones, and other important substances to the cells and organs in the body. This system also helps remove waste from the body.

Organs of the Cardiovascular System

Heart- Pumps blood throughout your body, provides needed oxygen to our organs and cells, and controls our heart rate and blood pressure.

Artery- Carries blood away from the heart and to the rest of the organs.

Veins- Carries blood toward the heart.

Capillaries (blood vessels)- Carries blood from arterioles to the venules. Assist with transportation of vital substances between the blood and tissue cells.

In proper balance:

Successful delivery of oxygen and nutrients to the cells and proper removal of waste.

Out of balance:

Oxygen and nutrients are not able to get to all the cells and thus cause aneurysm, lack of blood supply to the heart, chest pain, narrowed arteries, high blood pressure, clogged valves, and waste build-up.

Organ Affinity

Arjuna (Terminalia arjuna)
Coleus (Coleus forskohlii)
Curcumin (Curcumin longa)
Dong Quai (Angelica sinensis)
Hawthorn (Crataegus oxycantha)
Motherwort (Leonurus cardiaca)
Poke Root (Phytolacca america.)
Prickly Ash (Zanthoxylum ameri.)

System Actions

Cardiac Tonics
Circulatory Stimulants
Hemostatics
Hypotensives
Vasoconstrictors
Vasodilators

LYMPHATIC SYSTEM

The lymphatic system is part of the immune system. Its role is to protect the body from disease-causing organisms, maintain body fluid levels, fat transport, tissue drainage and removal of cell waste. The lymphatic systems move lymph fluids throughout the body. The lymph fluid (clear colorless fluid) contains vitamins, minerals, and nutrients, as well as bacteria, viruses, and damaged cells that may have entered the fluid. Lymph fluid only flows in an upward direction towards the neck.

Organs of the Lymphatic System

Lymphatic vessels- Transport's lymph fluid away from the tissues.

Lymph nodes- Filter out foreign substances, damaged cells and contains white blood cells that help fight infection.

Spleen- Filters your blood, protects bloodstream from bacterial and other infections. Controls the amount of red blood cells and the blood storage in the body.

Thymus- Make and train white blood cells called T Lymphocytes (T cells help fight infection).

Tonsils- Stops germs from entering in the mouth or nose.

Lymphatic tissue of the small intestines- Protects the body from invasion in the gut by regulating tissue fluid balance.

In proper balance:

Proper filtration of blood, production of antibodies, removal of toxic wastes. Maintains fluid levels in our body by balancing the fluid between our blood and tissues.

Out of balance:

Toxic waste gets backed up, weight loss, night sweats, fluid buildup in tissues, infections, cancers, and blockages.

Organ Affinity

Burdock (Arctium)
Marigold (Genus Tagetes)
Oregon Grape Root (Mahonia aquifol.)
Pipsessewa (Chimaphila)
Poke Root (Phytolacca americana)
Red Root (Ceanothus americanus)
Sarsaparilla (Smilax ornata)
Wild Indigo (Baptisia australis)

System Actions

Antioxidants
Detoxifers
Diaphoretics
Febrifuges
Immune Stimulants
Tonics

IMMUNE SYSTEM

The immune system is a powerful network made up of white blood cells, complement system, antibodies, lymphatic system, bone marrow, spleen and thymus. All of which work together to protect the body and to respond to threats.

Organs of the Immune System

Skin- One of the first lines of defense that protect you from pathogens (disease causing organisms).

Mucous Membranes- Layers of cells that surround all the body's entry points and organs (i.e., eyes, ears, and nose). Acts as a barrier by trapping foreign invaders.

Tonsils- Tonsils are covered with white blood cells to kill germs.

Thymus- Thymus provides surveillance and protection against pathogens.

Lymph Nodes- Filter out damaged cells and debris.

Spleen- Stores and filters blood and make white blood cells.

Bowel- 70% to 80% of your immune system is said to be housed in your gut. Processes our food and breaks down nutrients.

Bone Marrow- All the body's blood cells originate in the bone marrow. This is the main site for stem cell production.

In proper balance:

This system is able to protect us from infections and foreign invaders.

Out of balance:

Disorders of weakened immune system (acquired immune deficiency).

Overactive immune system (allergy).

Immune confusion (autoimmune disease).

Organ Affinity	System Actions
Ashwaganda (Withania somnifera)	Antibiotics
Astragalus (Astragalus membranaceus)	Febrifuges
Cedar (Thuja spp.)	Diaphoretics
Echinacea (Echinacea spp.)	Immunomodulator
Garlic (Allium sativa)	Immune Stimulants
Hyssop (Hyssopus Officinalis)	Tonics
Oregon Grape Root (Mahonia spp.)	
Wild Indigo (Baptsia tinctoria)	

RESPIRATORY SYSTEM

Consuming oxygen and producing carbon dioxide for the earth's atmosphere are necessary to life. The respiratory system is designed to eliminate carbon dioxide from the bloodstream and absorb oxygen from the earth's atmosphere. The respiratory system provides oxygen to the body's cells and removes carbon dioxide, a waste product, from the lungs through respiration (breathing).

Organs of the Respiratory System

Lungs- Brings in air from the atmosphere and moves oxygen into the blood stream.

Nose- Allows air to enter your body, filters debris and cleans the air you breathe.

Trachea (windpipe)- Carries air in and out of your lungs.

Throat (pharynx)- Carries air, food, and fluid from the nose and the mouth.

Voice box (larynx)- Allows speech and air into the lungs and blocks out food and other fluids.

Airways (bronchi)- Moves air to and from the lungs.

In proper balance:

The respiratory system can bring oxygen into our body (inspiration) and send out carbon dioxide (expiration) effectively. It will filter out dust and particles. The larynx can vibrate to make sounds.

Out of balance:

Inflamed airways, blood clots (stagnation in the blood), excess mucus, poor oxygen absorption, inflammation, fevers, respiratory infections, chills, muscle aches wheezing, coughing, and blockages in sinus openings.

Organ Affinity

Belladonna (Atropa belladonna)
Cloves (Syzygium aromaticum)
Cramp Bark (Viburnum)
Dong Quai (Angelica sinesis)
Mullein (Verbascum thapsus)
Oak (Quercus spp.)
Plantain (Plantago spp.)

System Actions

Antimicrobial
Antispasmodics
Astringents
Demulcents
Expectorants
Pectorals

DIGESTIVE SYSTEM

This system breaks down the food that you eat and moves it through your GI tract (stomach). What you eat is mixed with saliva and then moved into your stomach. The stomach releases digestive enzymes to help break down the food. The nutrients pass through your intestinal wall and enter your bloodstream. Once in the bloodstream, the nutrients are moved around the body to use for growth, cell repair, and energy. All non-absorbed food is moved to the colon and transformed into fecal matter to be removed.

Organs of the Digestive System

Mouth- Receives food and breaks it into smaller particles.

Esophagus- Carries food and liquid from your mouth to the stomach.

Stomach- Holds the food while enzyme acids break down food.

Salivary Glands- Make saliva to moisten food so it can be swallowed easily.

Liver- Filters the blood and makes bile.

Gallbladder- Store's the bile produced by the liver.

Pancreas- Contains enzymes that help you digest food and regulates blood sugar

Small intestine- Digests the food and absorbs nutrients.

Large intestine- Absorbs electrolytes, vitamins and water. Removes waste after all nutrients and vitamins have been disolved.

Anus- Controls the removal of feces.

In proper balance:

Your system can properly digest food, store and absorb nutrients and expel waste.

Out of balance:

Abdominal pain, diarrhea, bloating, indigestion, constipation, heartburn, ulcers, stomach acid leaks, inflammation of the stomach lining,

Organ Affinity

Boneset (Eupatorium perfoliatum)
Eucalyptus (Eucalyptus spp.)
Fennel (Foeniculum vulgare)
Fringe Tree (Chionanthus virginicus)
Ginger (Zingiber officinale)
Lungwort (Sticta pulmonaria)
Yellow Dock (Rumex spp.))

System Actions

Antimicrobials
Antispasmodics
Astringents
Bitters
Carminatives
Demulcents
Digestive Tonics
Hepatics
Laxatives
Sialagogues
Stomachics

URINARY SYSTEM

The main purpose of the urinary system is to get rid of wastes and excess water from the body, regulate the blood pH, control the levels of electrolytes and metabolites, and filter blood.

Organs of the Urinary System

Kidneys- Cleanses the blood of toxins, changes waste to urine, and removes excess fluid.
Ureters- Carries urine from kidneys and bladder.
Bladder- Stores the urine.
Urethra- Removes urine from the bladder to the outside of the body.

In proper balance:

The urinary system allows for proper filtration of waste products, proper regulation of water and salts, and contraction of bladder muscles.

Out of balance:

When the urinary system is out of balance it causes a build-up of waste substances, pain, bladder infections (UTI), inflammation, high fever, low back pain, kidney infections and stones, weak bladder, enlarged prostate.

Organ Affinity

Boneset (Eupatorium perfoliatum)
Burdock (Artium lappa)
Cleavers (Galium aparine)
Myrrh (Commiphora myrrha)
Oregano (Origanum vulgare)
Red Raspbery (Rubus idaeus)
Yarrow (Achillea millefolium)

System Actions

Antilithics
Diuretics
Kidney Tonics
Urinary Antiseptics
Urinary Astringents
Urinary Demulcents

REPRODUCTIVE SYSTEM FEMALE

A female system that comprises of tissues, organs and glands that are involved in the creation of children.

Organs of the Female Reproductive System

Ovaries- Produce eggs and hormones (estrogen and progesterone).

Cervix- Tube of tissue that connects the uterus to the vagina. Produces mucus and releases menstrual fluid during a period.

Uterus (womb)- Receives the fertilized egg and protects the fetus.

Fallopian Tubes- Transports sperm to the eggs and then transports the fertilized egg to the uterus.

Vagina- Provides a canal for sexual intercourse and childbirth.

In proper balance:

The body can produce gametes, produce egg cells necessary for reproduction, and shed uterine lining (menstrual flow).

Out of balance:

Imbalance results in infections, inflammation of the vagina, pain, scarring, cottage cheese discharge and high pH.

Organ Affinity

Black Cohosh (Actaea racemosa)
Black Haw (Viburnum prunifolium)
Bladderwrack (Fucus vesiculosus)
Chaste Tree (vitex agnus-castus)
Cramp Bark (Viburnum opulus)
Maca (Lepidium meyenii)
Nettles (Urtica dioica)

System Actions

Antispasmodics
Estrogenics
Oxytoxics
Uterine Tonics

REPRODUCTIVE SYSTEM: MEN

Male system that comprises of tissues, organs, and glands that are involved in the creation of children.

Organs of the Reproductive System Men

Ureter- Carries urine from the kidney to the bladder.

Prostate- Produces fluid for semen.

Testicles- Makes sperm and testosterone.

Urethra- Carries urine from bladder to the outside of the body. Releases semen during ejaculation.

Penis- Male sex organ. Is a conduit for urine to leave the body.

In proper balance:

The body can produce and transport sperm, regulates body temperature, and produce and secrete male sex hormones. Males will also experience a normal sex drive.

Out of balance:

Fatigue, low testosterone levels, low sperm count, low sex drive, impotence, and depression.

Organ Affinity	System Actions
Ashwaghanda (Withania somnifera)	Adaptogens
Ginkgo (Ginko biloba)	Antibacterial
Ginseng (Panax quinquefolia)	Anti parasitic
Nettles (Urtica dioica)	Anti-inflammatory
Oats (Avena sativa)	Blood Cleanser
Pygeum (Pygeum africanum)	Detoxifying
Saw Palmetto (Seronoa repens)	Tonics
Yohimbe (Pausinystalia yohimbe)	Urinary disinfectants

EXCRETORY SYSTEM

The excretory system is a system that removes excess, and unnecessary materials from our body fluids. This system helps to maintain internal chemical balance and prevent damage to our body.

Organs of the Excretory System

Skin- Skin sweats to eliminate excess water and salts, as well as a small amount of urea.

Liver- Breaks down many substances in the blood, including toxins. Transforms ammonia into urea so it can be filtered through the kidneys and removed through urine.

Large intestine- Eliminates solid wastes that linger after the digestion of food and collects wastes from throughout the body.

Lungs- A part of the respiratory system, responsible for the excretion of gaseous wastes from the body including carbon dioxide.

Kidneys- Eliminates excess water and wastes from the bloodstream by the production of the liquid waste known as urine.

In proper balance:

Wastes (ammonia, carbon dioxide, urea) and water is efficiently removed from the body.

Out of balance:

Toxic waste back up, weight loss, night sweats, fluid buildup in tissues, infections, cancers, and blockages.

Organ Affinity	System Actions
Aloe (Aloe vera)	Antiseptics
Black Haw (Viburnum prunifolium)	Antispasmodic
Corn silk (Zea Mays)	Demulcents
Dandelion (Taraxacum officinalis)	Diuretic
Goldenseal (Hyrastis canadensis)	Hepatic
Juniper Berry (Juniperus communis)	Hepatoprotective
Khella (Ammi visnaga)	Laxitive
Parsley (Petroselinum crispum)	Pectorals

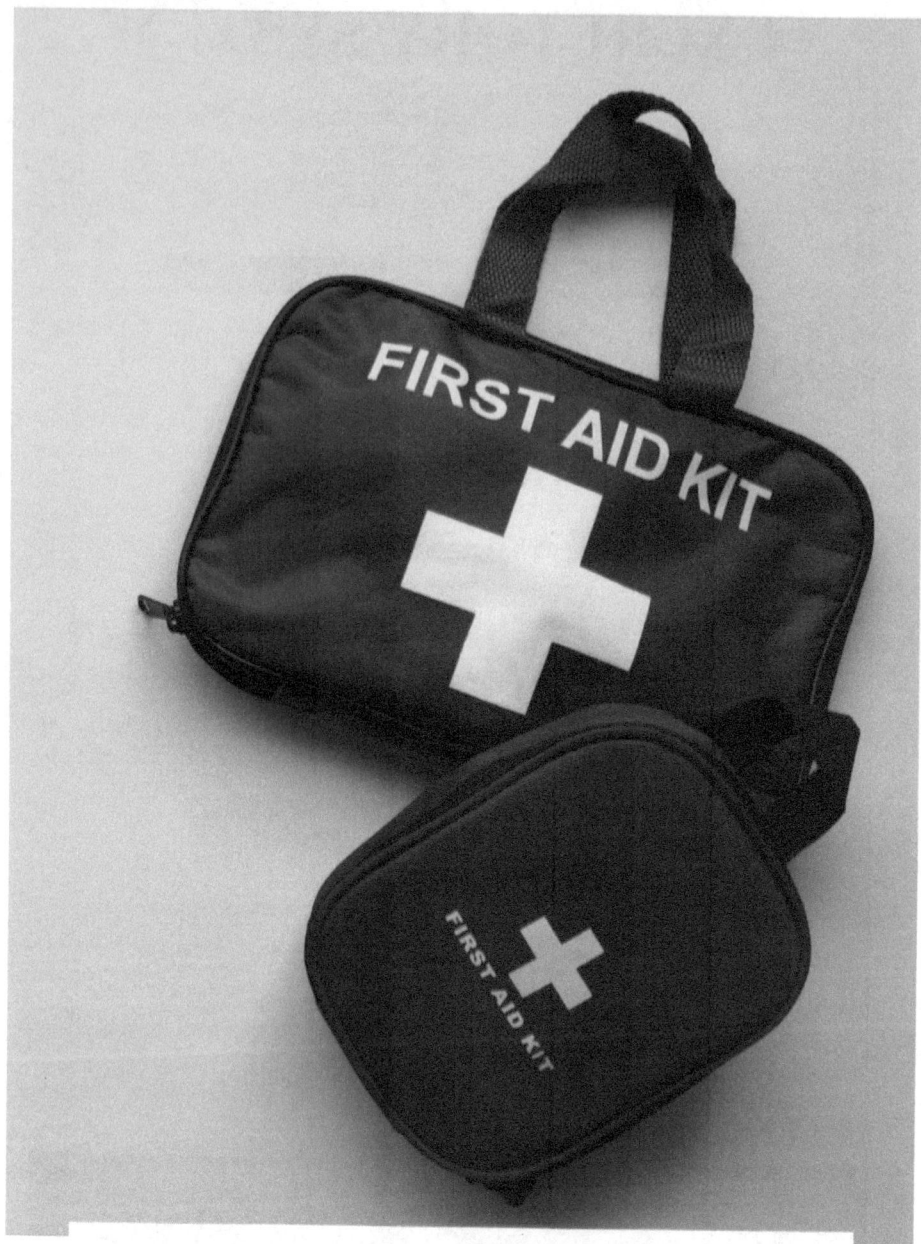

BASIC

FIRST AID

FIRST AID

Without proper First Aid, a simple injury could turn very serious or into a fatality. Death could occur as a result of lack of immediate medical treatment.

First Aid does not only promote a faster recovery, it helps save lives. Statistics from the Red Cross stated that about 60% of deaths from injuries could be prevented if first aid would have been offered before emergency medical services arrived at the scene.

Understanding the basic first aid procedures can help prevent a medical emergency from getting worse.

BLEEDING

Make sure to first wash your hands and put on protective gloves to create barrier between you and the victim. Also cleanse your hands thoroughly with soap and water when finished.

Basic first aid treatment:

- CALL 911 for medical assistance.
- Keep victim lying down.
- Apply direct pressure to the wound by using a clean cloth or sterile dressing.
- If there is an object lodged in a wound, do not try to remove it. See a doctor to help remove it.
- Check for fractures, if there are none, carefully elevate the wound above the victim's heart.
- Once you control the bleeding, keep victim warm by covering with a blanket. Monitor for shock.

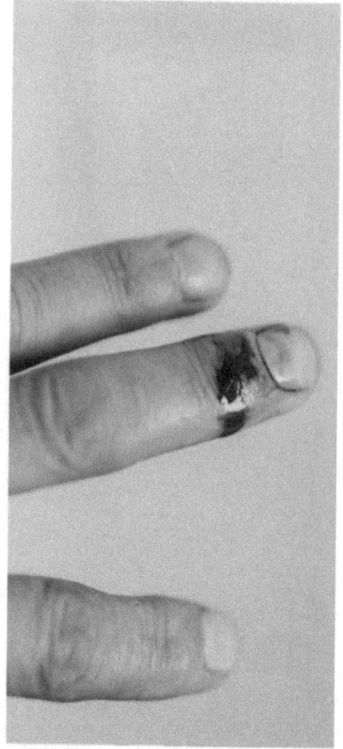

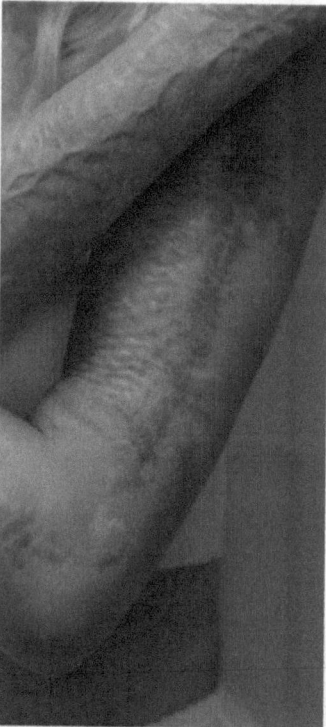

BURNS

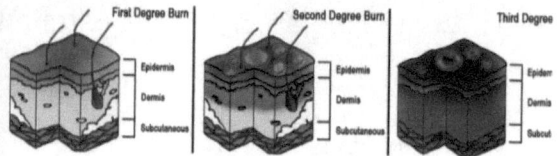

Image: Persian Poet Gal at English Wikipedia, CC BY 3.0

1st degree & some 2nd degree burns:

- Submerge burn area in cool water to stop the pain. If the impacted area is large, cover the person with cool, wet cloths. If pain persists but no medical assistance is needed, then apply medicated first aid cream/gel and cover burn with a sterile dressing.
- If the person needs medical attention cover burn with a dry, sterile dressing, no creams/gels, and seek medical help immediately.
- For 3rd degree & certain 2nd degree burns: CALL 911!! Third degree burns have to receive medical care and must be done immediately. Do not remove clothes that are stuck to the burn.

INFANT CHOKNG

- Place infant facing downward on your forearm supporting their head and neck with your hand.
- Place your hand on your knee with the infant's head lower than it's body.
- Use the heel of your hand give four strong blows on the infants back between the it's shoulder blades.
- Then turn the infant over, place two fingers on the center of the infant's chest (just below the nipples) and perform up to five chest thrusts.
- Repeat until the obstruction is clear.
- Take the infant to get medical attention after any choking incident, incase any complications arise.

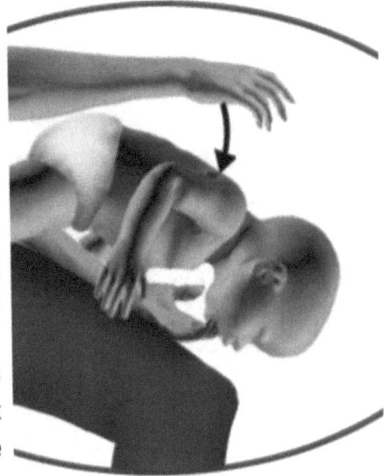

Image: BruceBlaus, CC BY-SA 4.0 via Wikimedia Commons

UNCONSCIOUSNESS

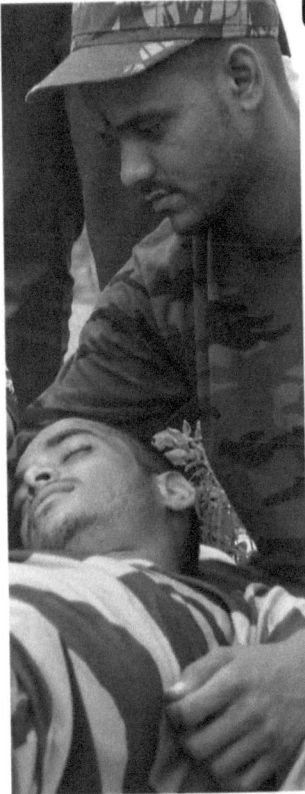

- Do not leave an unconscious victim alone unless you are calling 911 for help.
- Check if the person is aware by asking if they are OK.
- Check their Airway, Breathing, and Circulation (ABC's).
- If the victim's ABC's are not present, perform CPR.
  - **CPR**: Call 911 or ask someone else to.
  - Lay the person on their back and open their airway.
  - Check for breathing.
  - Perform 30 chest compressions.
  - Perform two rescue breaths.
  - Repeat until medical help or automated external defibrillator (AED) arrives.
- If ABC's are there and there is no suspected spinal injury, place the person on their side with their chin toward the ground to allow for fluid drainage.
- Cover the person a with blanket to keep them warm and prevent shock. Take it off if they get hot.

CHOKING

- First ask the person, "Are you OK?"
- If the person cannot speak, breathe, or cough, ask a nearby person to call 911 and begin performing the Heimlich maneuver (abdominal thrust).
- Get behind the person with your arms around their stomach. Place your thumb-side of your fist above the persons navel and below the lower end of the breastbone. Grab your fist with your free hand and pull your fist upward and in, quickly and firmly.
- Continue with thrusts until the object is dislodged or airway is clear.

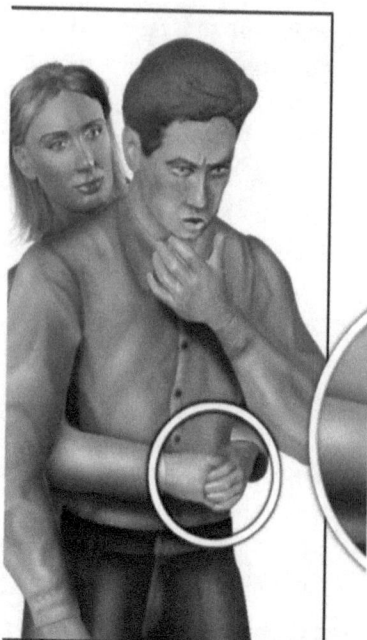

Image: BruceBlaus, CC BY-SA 4.0 via Wikimedia Commons

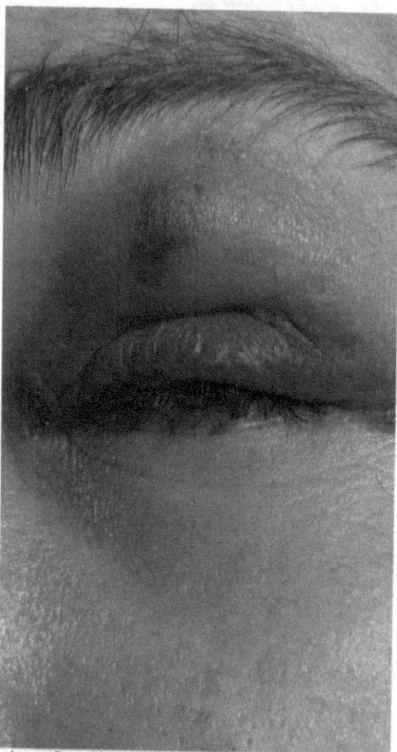

Image: BruceBlaus, CC BY-SA 4.0 via Wikimedia Commons

EYE INJURY'S

- If an object is impaled in the eye, CALL 911 and DO NOT try to remove the object.
- Use sterile dressings to cover both eyes. This will prevent further injury.
- DO NOT rub or apply pressure, raw meat, or ice to the injured eye.
- For a black eye, you can apply ice to cheek and the area around eye.

How to flush the eyes:

If chemical is in only one eye, flush by turning the persons head with the contaminated eye downward to prevent contaminating the other eye. Flush with cool or room temperature water for 15 minutes or more.

If applicable, remove contact lenses after you flush the eyes.

S U R V I V E

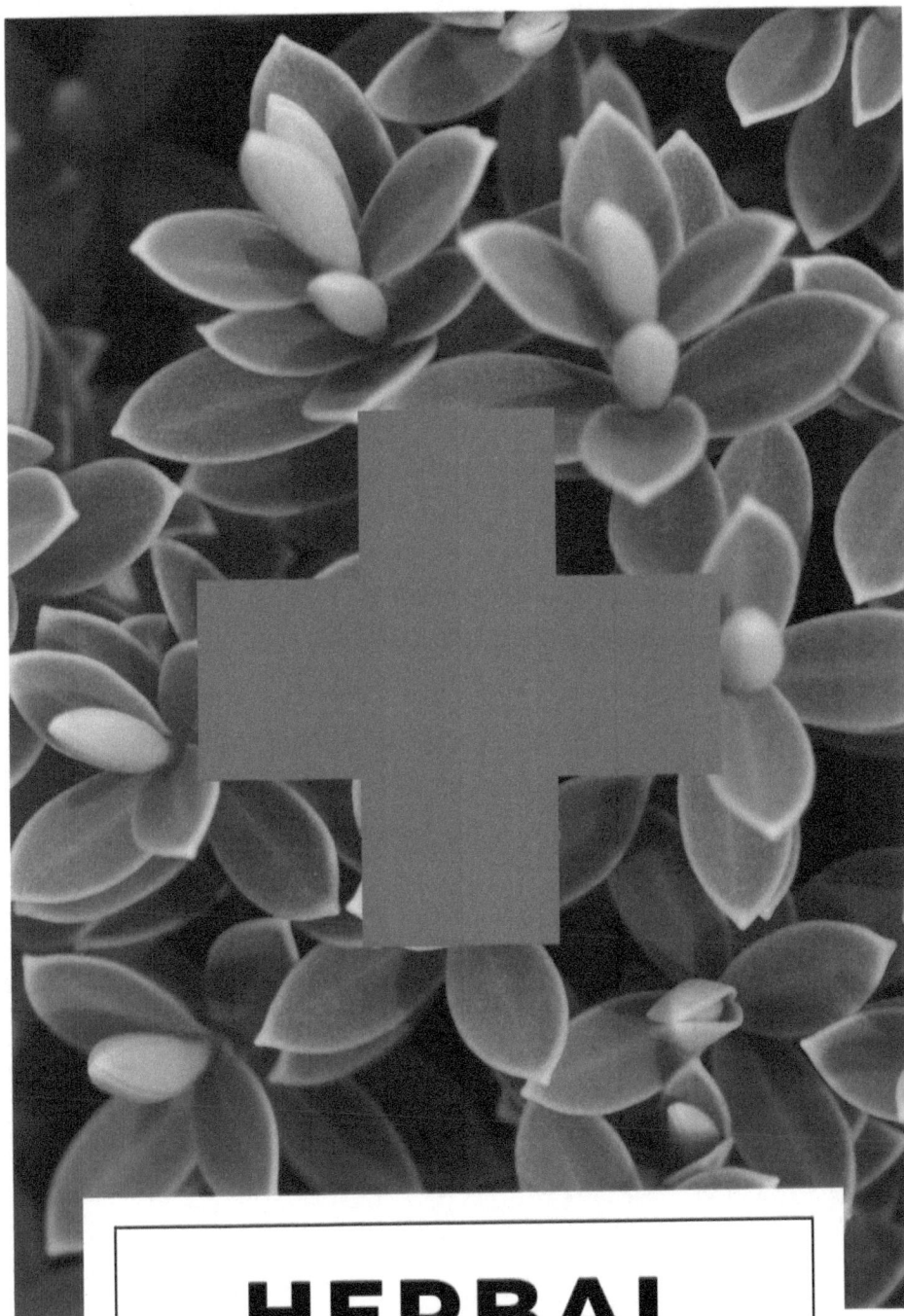

HERBAL

FIRST AID

HERBAL FIRST AID?

Herbal First Aid is imply using herbs to address many first aid situations that you might find yourself in. You can either make the remedies yourself or purchase them from an herbalist product creator. The ideal situation is for you to know about these common issues and the formulas that can help you address them. This is in the event that no one is around to help you. It is important to be able to positively identify common weeds and herbs that grow around you around you so the medicine will be handy in case of emergency.

In your herbal first aid kit be sure to have a book filled with the phone numbers of emergency medical staff, local hospitals, poison control and trauma centers. Also note the location of nearest radio or telephone, and emergency dentist.

When creating your own herbal first aid products consider the therapeutic categories for each first aid situation and determine which herbal medicines you have to address them.

HERBS FOR FIRST AID

- Aloe- Aloe vera
- Anemone–Anemone spp.
- Arnica–Arnica spp.
- Astragalus–Astragalus spp.
- Balsam Gum- Abies balsamea (L.)
- Black cohosh–Actaea racemosa
- Black Haw- Viburnum prunifolium
- Blue vervain–Verbena hastata
- Boneset- Eupatorium perfoliatum
- Calendula–Calendula officinalis
- California poppy–Eschscholzia spp.
- Catnip–Nepeta cataria
- Cayenne–Capsicum annuum
- Chamomile–Matricaria chamomilla
- Chaparral–Larrea tridentata
- Chickweed–Stellaria media
- Comfrey–Symphytum spp.
- Conifer resin–various species
- Creosote Bush-Larrea tridentata
- Damiana–Turnera diffusa
- Echinacea–Echinacea spp.
- Elder- Sambucus nigra
- Flowering Dogwood
- Garlic–Allium sativum
- Ghost pipe–Monotropa uniflora
- Ginger–Zingiber officinale
- Goldenseal–Hydrastis canadensis
- Gotu kola–Centella asiatica
- Hops–Humulus lupulus
- Jamaican dogwood–Piscidia piscipula
- Jewelweed- Impatiens capensis
- Joe Pye Weed- Eutrochium purpu.
- Kava kava–Piper methysticum
- Licorice–Glycyrrhiza spp.
- Lobelia–Lobelia inflata
- Marijuana–Cannabis spp.
- Marshmallow–Althaea officinalis
- Meadowsweet–Filipendula ulmaria
- Motherwort–Leonurus cardiaca
- Mustard–Brassica spp.
- Myrrh–Commiphora myrrha
- Neem- Azadirachta indica
- Nettles–Urtica dioica
- Oak–Quercus spp.
- Oregon graperoot–Berberis spp.
- Osha–Ligusticum porteri
- Passionflower–Passiflora incarnata
- Pennyroyal- Mentha pulegium
- Plantain–Plantago spp.
- Poplar–Populus spp.
- Prickly ask–Zanthoxylum spp.
- Propolis–Bee resin
- Quinine Bush- Cinchona pubescens
- Red Clover- Trifolium pratense
- Reishi–Ganoderma spp.
- Sarsaparilla- Smilax officinalis
- Shepherd's purse–Capsella bursa.
- Silk tassel–Garrya spp.
- Skullcap–Scutellaria lateriflora
- Slippery elm–Ulmus rubra
- St. John's wort–Hypericum perforatum
- Sweet Flag- Acorus calamus
- Tea–Camellia sinensis
- Tea Tree- Melaleuca alternifolia
- Tulsi–Ocimum tenuiflorum
- Turmeric–Curcuma longa
- Valerian–Valeriana officinalis
- White Pine- Pinus strobus
- Wild lettuce–Lactuca spp.
- Wild Pansy- Viola tricolor
- Wild Yam- Dioscorea villosa
- Willow–Salix spp.
- Witch hazel–Hamamelis virginiana
- Yarrow–Achillea millefolium
- Yerba del mansa–Anemopsis californica

HERB ACTIONS

These categories group herbal medicines based on similar therapeutic actions. This will help you to know exactly what herb you can use to target the specific first aid issue. Keep in mind that some plants might fit into one or more categories so this can lessen the amount of herbs that you put into your formulations.

Adsorbent—Attracts and holds foreign material.
Anesthetic—Reduces local sensation.
Antibacterial- Effects against a variety of bacteria.
Anti Viral- Herbs that slow or stop the replication of invading viruses.
Anti fungal- Address fungal infections.
Anti-inflammatory—Reduces inflammation.
Anti-lithics- Herbs that prevent formation of calculi or stones.
Antimicrobial—Inhibits or kills microorganisms.
Antiseptic—Topical antimicrobial agent.
Antispasmodics- Relax Muscles .
Anxiolytic—Reduces anxiety.
Astringent—Constricts and tightens body tissues, reduces discharges.
Bitters- Stimulate the digestive tract.
Carminatives- Relieves belching. flatus and bloating.
Circulatory stimulants—Stimulates circulation.
Demulcent—Soothes mucous membranes often with a mucilaginous texture.
Emetics- Induces vomiting.
Emollient—Skin softening, a moisturizer.
Expectorants- Liquefy hard phlegm and moves wastes from respiratory system.
Febrifuges- Help eliminate toxins and address the issues that cause a high fever.
Hemostatic—Stops bleeding.
Immunostimulants—Increase various immune system components.
Laxatives- Helps you go to the bathroom.
Nervines- Herbs that restore and balance the nervous system.
Pain relievers—General pain reliever.
Relaxants- Mild relaxation action.
Rubefacient—Stimulates local blood vessels causing skin reddening.
Sedative—Calms and reduces excitability, tranquilizing.
Sleep aid—Helps with sleeping.
Trauma aid—Helps with recovery from shock and trauma.
Urinary Antiseptics- Disinfect the urinary tract.
Vulnerary—Wound healing agent.

ISSUES THAT HERBS CAN ADDRESS

- Skin injuries: Cuts, burns, scrapes, punctures, sprains, strains,
- Contusions
- Splinters
- Anemia
- Insect bites
- Dermatitis, Rashes, sunburn
- Asthma and Anaphylaxis
- Stomach Issues (diarrhea, constipation, viral gastroenteritis, parasites)
- Female issues (cramps, flooding, pregnancy, mastitis, menopause, prostatitis)
- Eye Issues (injuries or styes)
- Dental Issues (teething, abscess, crack or loss)
- Frost bite.
- Urinary System Issues (Kidney, Bladder, Urinary Tract Infection)
- Emotional/Psychiatric (anxiety, panic attacks, organizer-overwhelm)
- Circulatory Issues, Edema
- Scrapes, bruises, cuts
- Digestive upset (nausea, cramping, etc)
- Cold / Flu/ cough symptoms
- Fluids to relieve heat stress or dehydration
- Headaches (including migraines)
- Pain, cramps, muscle spasms, etc.
- Minor burns (including blisters and sunburn)
- Shock
- Herpes outbreaks
- Respiratory disorders

ISSUES THAT NEED MORE THAN HERBS CAN ADDRESS

Herbs can do some amazing things. However there are some conditions that cannot be treated by herbs alone. In this case, there is a time when a person will need to seek additional medical care. The following information is outlining situations that occur that will cause a person to seek medical care.

- If injury is beyond what you are capable of and your experience.
- If the pain is substantial and/or constant.
- If there is substantial bruising.
- If your wound needs stitches.

Red Flag Signs and Safety Concerns

If you see any of the following signs or symptoms, call 911 immediately. This list is not exhaustive.

- Uncontrolled bleeding
- Pains in their chest
- Loss of sensation anywhere in the body
- Pain in the spinal after a fall.
- Person lost consciousness or responsiveness
- Suspected bone fractures (pain won't stop after 20 minutes).
- Partial or full thickness burns
- Any type of Snake or animal bites
- Asthma attacks that are unresponsive to treatment or medications
- Suspected stroke or heart attack
- Person experiences a seizures of unknown origin
- Severe allergic reactions
- Persistent, localized, or severe abdominal pain.
- Fevers that are associated with severe headache or stiff neck
- Quick and sharp headaches.
- Diarrhea or vomit with blood in it.
- Person is unable to hydrate.

Other signs or symptoms of serious injury

Have faith in the plants, however, call 9-1-1 or take the person to the hospital or clinic needed and you are unsure with what to do.

HERBAL FIRST AID KIT

There is no one size fits all approach to how you put your herbal first aid kit together. Some people maybe dealing with different issues that cause a need for a particular remedy. For example, someone might regularly deal with digestive issues. This means that they need to have a digestive support remedy in their herbal first aid kit. Another person might have a kid that has eczema. So this person might consider a healing and cooling salve to address the scars/wounds. As you can see how you put together your kit is very personalized. I will tell you some of the main components that you might want to consider adding.

Herbal First Aid Kit Essentials
- Basic First Aid Kit
- Salves and liniments (wound, bruise, dry skin, sores)
- Herbal Bug Spray
- Tinctures (Pain relief, stomach relief, antiseptic, sedative, stress/anxiety, build immune system, constipation, sleep aid, increase circulation)
- Resins (wound healing, antiseptics)
- Compresses (wounds, burns)
- Herbal Powders (for compresses, bleeding, and poultices)
- Infused oils (ear aches, stress relief, bug bites)
- Lozenges and drops (shock, trauma, respiratory issues, nausea, motion sickness, throat issues)
- Washes (wounds, eyes)
- Herbal Plasters
- Capsules (empty and pre-mixed, ginger, turmeric, activated charcoal, etc.)
- Honey
- Ginger (dried and powdered)
- Tea bags (eye issues, digestive issues)
- Activated Charcoal
- Tea tree oil
- Lavender Essential Oil
- Top 10 essential oils
- 2 Carrier oils
- Extra mini glass bottles for on the spot blending
- Recipe cards for popular and necessary blends.
- List of herbs in your area and where to find them
- Stationary: pencils, pens, paper
- Pipettes and cloths for poultices and compresses

GOOD SAMARITAN LAWS

When you see a person who is in distress and might need first aid, don't let your fear of getting sued get in the way of you helping them. There is a law that can protect you. Its called the Good Samaritan Law.

Good Samaritan Laws are state laws also known as "volunteer protection laws." They are enacted to protect healthcare providers and other rescue personnel from being sued as a result of providing help to a victim during an emergency situation. Essentially they provide legal immunity if a person chooses to help. Vermont's Good Samaritan Law is unique in the USA and actually orders citizens to help fellow humans in need!

Check the laws in your state to see what your limitations might be.

METHODS TO ADMINISTER HERBS

PREPARATION DESCRIPTIONS

How you give your herbal remedy to someone is important. Not all methods of administration is appropriate for all herbal remedies. Some remedies are best administered as a tincture and others in an herbal pill form. Here are some of the ways you can administer your herbal remedies.

Compress- A cloth soaked in a strong tea and applied topically.

Creams- Water, carrier oils and essential oils.

Decoctions- Herbs placed in water and boiled for a specified time.

Essential oil- Concentrated aromatic oils distilled from plants.

Infused oil- Plant prepared in a fixed oil (i.e., coconut oil, for external use).

Liniment- Plants prepared in isopropyl (rubbing) alcohol (for external use).

Medicinal Wines- Soaking herbs in rice, sorghum wine, other alcohol.

Ointments- Steeping herbs in a carrier oil (oil or beeswax).

Poultice- Plants cut up and/or cooked and applied topically.

Powder- Plants ground into powder form.

Salve- An infused oil with beeswax added.

Soak- A strong tea where the body part is placed directly in the fluid

Syrups- Decocted herbs in steeped in sugar or honey.

Tea- Plants prepared in water.

Tincture- Plants prepared in ethanol (drinking alcohol)

Washes- Herbs infused in rose water, aloe etc.

COMPRESS

A compress is similar to a poultice in that we are applying plant products to the skin, but instead of applying plant material directly to the skin, we are applying a cloth that has been soaked in a strong herbal infusion or decoction.

Issues a compress addresses:
Hemorrhoids, sore muscles, internal congestion, bruises, inflammation, acute burns.

Best part of the plant to use:
Roots, barks, seed, flowers, leaves

Supplies needed to prepare:

- Quart-Sized Pot with Lid
- Herbs
- Fine-Mesh Strainers (unbleached cheesecloth)
- Cloth

Simple recipe:
- Bring water to boil in a heavy pot.
- Infuse/decoction herbs in water.
- Add the herbs to the water and reduce heat so that the water is simmering.
- Leave the herbs to simmer gently for 15 to 20 minutes.
- Strain out the herbs and collect the tea.
- Soak the cloth in the tea and then wring out the cloth.
- Secure it on the affected area

Recommended dosage:
For the majority of commonly used herbs, the range is 6-15 grams for a one day dose, with an average of about 10 grams/day.

CREAMS

Infused oils are made by steeping herbs in a carrier oil like olive or almond to extract the medicinal plant constituents that will help soothe your skin.

What issues are best addressed with creams:

Cracked dry skin, bug bites, burns, chapped skin, abrasions, sunburns, hives and hangnails.

Best Part of the plant to use:
Flowers, Roots, Leaves

Supplies Needed:

- 1/4 cup butter (shea, mango, cocoa)
- 1/8 cup carrier oil (olive, almond, apricot)
- 1 tablespoon beeswax
- 10 drops essential oil 1
- 10 drops essential oil 2

Simple Recipe:

- Melt the butters, beeswax, and carrier oils together in a double boiler.
- Mix until they melt and mix together.
- After everything is melted remove it from heat and allow it to cool for 5-10 minutes.
- Put in the essential oils and pour the cream into glass containers.
- Allow to harden completely (can take several hours).

Storage:

Store the homemade hand cream at room temperature for up to 3 months, away from direct sunlight, heat and moisture.

Recommended Dosage:

Apply this cream to your dry hands as often as needed.

DECOCTIONS

A decoction is an herbal preparation created by boiling herbs in liquid. They are more concentrated than herbal infusions.

What issues are best addressed with decoctions?

- Acute conditions (short duration illnesses)

Best Part of the plant to use?

- Stems, Roots, Bark and Rhizome

Supplies needed to prepare

- Quart-Sized Pot with Lid
- Reusable Tea Bags or Unbleached Disposable Tea Filter Bags
- Fine-Mesh Strainers (unbleached cheesecloth)
- Quart-Sized Glass Jars

Simple Recipe

1. Bring water to boil in a heavy pot.
2. Measure herbs. Use approximately 1 teaspoon of dried (or 2 teaspoons of fresh) herbs per 1 cup of water.
3. Add the herbs to the water and reduce heat so that the water is simmering.
4. Leave the herbs to simmer gently for 15 to 20 minutes.
5. Strain out the herbs.

Recommended Dosage

For the majority of commonly used herbs, the range is 6-15 grams for a one day dose, with an average of about 10 grams/day. Use approximately 1 teaspoon of dried or 2 teaspoons of fresh herbs per 1 cup of water.

HAND ROLLED PILLS

Herb pills herb powder with honey and rolling into a pill. Typically, these pills were made with one-third honey and two-thirds herb powder, and the pill size was about 6 or 9 grams total.

What issues are best addressed with Pills:
Herbal pills can be used to addressed a variety of issues.

Best Part of the plant to use:
Roots, Flowers, Leaves

Supplies needed:
- Raw herbs
- Honey
- Glass jar
- Knife
- Cutting board

Simple Recipe:
1. Start with a blend of finely powdered herbs.
2. Add a 1 tbsp of raw honey and enough water until the mix resembles bread dough.
3. Split your dough into two or three pieces and roll them into a long thin rope.
4. Cut the rope into small pieces.
5. Roll each segment into pea-sized balls or smaller.
6. Coat each ball in a powder of your choice (cinnamon, cocoa, etc.) and refrigerate in a glass jar until needed.

Storage
When stored in a dry place out of direct sunlight, rolled herb pills should have a shelf-life of 3 months or so. Refrigerating them can help extend their shelf-life, but keep in mind that the more time passes, the less effective the pills will be

Expiration: Capsule supplements are stable and potent if properly maintained for two to three years, but this depends on the product.

Dosage:
The dose would usually be one pill each time, one to three times per day depending on the condition. Thus, the dosing would typically range from 12-18 grams of the herb powder.

INFUSED OILS

Herbal infusions are made from the infusion herbs, spices, or other plant material in a carrier oil.

What issues are best addressed with infusions?

Skin issues, bacterial or viral issues.

Best Part of the plant to use:

Roots, Shoots, Leaves, and Flowers

Option 1: Simple Recipe (cold infusion)

1. Scoop dried herbs into a dark glass jar.
2. Cover herbs with carrier oil.
3. Shake the jar and place in a cool area for 2-4 weeks.

Supplies needed to prepare

- Dried herb of your choice.
- Carrier oil (olive, coconut etc.)
- Glass jar with a tight lid

Option 2: Heat Infusion

1. Place herbs in crock-pot or double boiler and cover with carrier oil of choice, leaving at least an inch or two of oil above your herbs.
2. Heat the herbs over very low heat (between 100° and 140° F) for approximately 1 to 5 hours or until the oil takes on the color and scent of the herb.
3. Turn off heat and allow to cool.
4. Once oil is cooled, strain the oil using a cheesecloth.
5. Then place in a dry and sterilized glass bottle.
6. Label your bottles with the date and product contents before storing them.
7. Store in a cool, dark, dry place for up to six months. You can add Vitamin E oil to prolong shelf life for oils to be used on top of our skin.

LINIMENTS

A liniment is an herbal remedy that is used topically to help alleviate pain in sore muscles and soft tissues. It's made with either rubbing alcohol or witch hazel, allowing the herbs can be easily and quickly absorbed into the skin.

What issues are best addressed with herbal liniments?
Pain in sore muscles and soft tissues.

Best Part of the plant to use?
Roots, Leaves, Flowers

Supplies Needed:
- Rubbing Alcohol or witch hazel
- Fresh or dried herbs.
- Optional additions: Essential oil(s) of choice.

Recipe
1. Chop herbs and put in a clean glass jar.
2. Cover the herbs with rubbing alcohol or witch hazel and put a tightly fitting cap on.
3. Place the jar in a warm area and shake daily or as often as possible for 4 to 6 weeks.
4. After 4-6 weeks, use cheese cloth to strain the herbs out.
5. If desired, add essential oil(s). Then pour the liniment into your dark glass bottles.

Storage:
When properly stored in a cool dark place, the liniment will keep almost indefinitely.

Recommended Dosage
As needed, but no more than 3 to 4 times a day.

MEDICINAL WINES

Medicinal wine is an alcoholic drink produced by soaking herbs in rice wine or grain alcohol.

What issues are best addressed with Medicinal Wines?
Wine is known as the "strength of a hundred medicines." Medicinal wines prevent and treat disorders and promote longevity. Blood stasis, meridian obstruction, and/or cold syndrome: arthritis, diuretic and febrifuge (to reduce fever) and to treat many different ailments, including anxiety, eye pain, obstinate ulcers, and head wounds.

Best Part of the plant to use?
leaves, roots, bark, fruit, seeds, flowers.

Simple Recipe
- For every pint of wine, use approximately 1 ounce of dried herbs and/or spices.
- Put the herbs in the bottle or jar and pour the wine over.
- Cap this tightly and shake well.
- Store the infusing jars in a cool place, out of direct light.
- They should be shaken up every day or so for 1-3 weeks. After that, strain the herbs using a strainer and several layers of clean cheesecloth, and return to a clean jar or a bottle.

Supplies needed to prepare
- Wine (red and white wines make for delicious concoctions)
- Glass Jar
- Herbs and Spices
- Strainer

Storage:
The wine can last for up to two weeks once infused. The wines should store for a few months if they are well-capped.

Recommended Dosage
Dosage: 1 Tablespoon to a 1/2 cup each day.

OINTMENTS

Ointments are semisolid preparations applied to the skin, eyes, and mucus membranes. Ointments can be used for medicinal purposes that can either act on the skin or be absorbed through the skin to act on our systems.

What issues are best addressed with herbal ointment?

to use on bites, stings, bumps,hemorrhoids, bruises, burns, and clean scrapes and cuts.

Best Part of the plant to use?

Roots, Leaves, Stem

Supplies Needed:

- Handful of fresh Herb 1 (your choice)
- Handful of fresh Herb 2 (your choice)
- Handful of fresh Herb 3 (your choice)
- 1 1/4 cup carrier oil
- 1 ounce beeswax (by weight)
- 40 drops essential oil (optional)
- Tins or containers.

Simple Recipe

1. Chop herbs
2. Place the wilted and finely chopped plants in the top of a double boiler (or a bowl placed over a pot). Pour in the oil.
3. Heat the oil via the double boiler. Keep the temperature around 100° F.
4. Strain off the plant material and measure out 1 cup of oil.
5. On low heat, heat the beeswax. Once it has melted then add the herb oil and stir. Stir until everything is melted down and combined.
6. Remove from heat. Add the essential oils. Stir well. Then pour mixture into your containers

Recommended Dosage

Adults and children 1 year of age and over—Apply to affected area(s) of the skin three or four times a day.

Storage:

Store out of direct sunlight and in a cool dry place free from moisture.

PLANT BASED SOAPS
Plants that Can be Used as Soap!

What are saponins?

Saponins are steroids that dissolve in water and create a stable froth. Saponins are named from the Soapwort plant (Saponaria) whose roots were used historically as soap. The fruits of several native North American plants contain high levels of saponins to produce lather and can be used as soaps or shampoos.

This group of plants includes:

- Atriplex roots (Atriplex hortensis),
- Sapindus fruits (Sapindus saponaria),
- Mojave yucca root (Yucca schidiger),
- Soapwort root (European species), and
- Buffalo berry fruits (Shepherdia argentea).

Natural Soap Plants:

Missouri gourd (Cucurbita foetidissima) Used as a shampoo, hand and laundry soap.

Wild lilac (Ceanothus)- Flowers lather and create soaps.

California soap plant (Chlorogalum pomeridianum)- Bulbs create the soap.

Soap Berry(Sapindus)- Boil to create soap

Soapweed yucca (Yucca glauca) Yucca roots has a high concentration of saponins and can be used for soap and shampoo. The lathering substances called saponins are found in many plants, but are exceptionally concentrated in yucca roots.

Buffalo Berry (Shepherdia rotundifolia)- Has uses for saponins. The high levels of saponin make it best for creating soaps, natural cleansing products, and shampoo.

Soapwort (Saponaria officinalis)- Used in some gentle skin cleaning products.

Soap plant (Chlorogalum pomeridianum)-The fibrous bulb with a white 'heart' inside, produces soapy substance when its crushed. It can be used as a conditioner and laundry soap for delicate fabrics. It is also used as soap.

Clematis (Clematis)-Collect the leaves and flowers. Crush and boil them to get a soapy solution.

Horse Chestnut(Aesculus hippocastanum)- Saponin rich seeds produce a rich lather when you rub seeds in the palm of your hands. You can also keep the crushed seed in water overnight to obtain a milky solution, which you can use as a detergent.

POULTICES

A poultice is the direct application of the fresh herb to the skin.

What issues are best addressed with compresses and poultices?
Poultices are primarily used short term for wounds, skin issues, injuries, pain, splinters, insect bites and stings, nettle stings, inflammation, spider bites, bruises, sprains, a rash, dry skin, a burn, or strains.

Types of Poultices

- **Drawing poultices**: Used to draw a foreign object to the surface of the skin so it can be removed. Use drawing herbs, charcoal, baking soda, and/or clay powders. Used to address splinters, insect bites and stings, nettle stings, spider bites, etc. Use herbs have an anti-inflammatory, pain-relieving.

- **Soothing poultices**: Used to soothe the skin. Made with anti-inflammatory, analgesic, vulnerary, and cooling herbs, honey, etc. They are indicated for such things as bites and stings, rashes, sunburns, dry skin, and itching.

- **Stimulating poultices**: Used to increase circulation. Made with warming, analgesic, or anti-inflammatory herbs. Stimulating poultices are used to help increase circulation to an area and herbs that have rubefacient qualities or that are warming in nature.

- **Pain relieving poultices**: Used to ease aches and pains (e.g. sore muscles, cramping, strains, sprains, ear aches, etc.), made with analgesic, antispasmodic, and anti-inflammatory herbs

Best Part of the plant to use for poultices?
Roots, Barks and Seeds

Supplies needed to prepare
- Fresh Herbs (flowers, leaves, stems, roots (in powder form))
- Warm Water
- Wrap with gauze or muslin

Simple Recipe
- Mash herbs into a paste
- Apply paste to effected area
- Secure the poultice in place with bandage or cloth

Recommended Dosage
Poultices can be applied for a very short period – sometimes 10 to 30 minutes is enough or they can be applied and left overnight or re-applied as needed throughout the day.

POWDERS

Herbal Powders come from different herbs dried and grounded into a powder. Herbal powders are perfect for making cordials, syrups, or wine.

What issues are best addressed with Herbal powders:
Powders help in condition the hair and nourish the scalp. Powders can also boost immunity, purify the blood, and relieve joint and muscle pain.

Best Part of the plant to use:
Roots, Flowers, Stems

Supplies needed to prepare:

- Blender
- Coffee Mill
- Bowl
- Mesh Strainers
- Herbs
- Roots, leaves, and flowers.

Simple Recipe:

- Grind the herbs.
- Mix the powdered herbs and powder base in a bowl,breaking up any clumps.
- Pass powdered herbs through a fine mesh strainer to remove any large particles.
- Store in a shaker or glass jar

Recommended Dosage:
Today, various sources suggest a range of dosages from 3 g to 18 g per day. You can use larger dosages for acute (short-term) conditions and smaller doses for chronic (long-term) conditions, especially when deficiency is involved, and long-term therapy is needed.

SALVES

A salve is a medical ointment used to soothe the surface of the body.

What issues are best addressed with salves?

Painful scrapes, itchy rashes, dry and irritated skin, muscle and joints, aches and pains, dull skin complexion issues such as pimples and blackheads, as well as scalp conditions, such as ringworm. Chapped lips, and even diaper rash. Salves also work to help soothe sunburn, eczema, and cuts.

Best Part of the plant to use:

Flowers, Leaves, and Roots

Supplies needed to prepare:

- Double Boiler Set Up
- Containers Liquid Measuring Cup
- Sack Cloths & Fine Mesh Sieve
- Silicone scraper or spatula
- Carrier Oils (coconut, olive, sesame, safflower, sweet almond oil)
- Waxes (beeswax, carnuba)
- Herbs

Simple Recipe:

- 1 cups base oil blend of your choice I like coconut oil and olive oil here
- ½ cup dried herb(s) of your choice
- 2-4 tablespoon beeswax pastilles
- Essential oil of your choice see dilution ratios in post

Instructions:

1. Infuse your herbs into the base oils then strain through layers of sack cloth squeeze to extract all the oil.
2. Pour infused to a double boiler, add your beeswax and warm until completely melted (add more beeswax as needed for thicker consistency.)
3. Remove mixture from heat, add essential oils, and mix.
4. Pour mixture into individual 2-ounce containers (about 4) or other similarly sized jars. Allow to cool completely before putting a lid on the container.
5. Use within a year.

Expiration

Your salve should last you about 6 months (twice as long if refrigerated).

SYRUPS

Herbal infused syrups are concentrated herbal teas, preserved in sugar or honey. They are an alternative to alcohol-based tinctures for children or people avoiding alcohol.

What issues are best addressed with Syrups?
Respiratory issues, Cold and Flu's

Best Part of the plant to use?
Heavier plant parts, roots, stems, dense roots, berries and barks need to be simmered longer anyways.

Supplies needed:
- Herbs
- Water
- Honey
- Glass jars
- Boiling pot

Simple Recipe
The basic recipe for an herbal syrup:
1 cup of herb
2 – 3 cups of water
1 – 1.5 cups of honey

Directions:
1. Make a very strong decoction, using 1 ounce of herb per 16 ounces of water. Warm the herbs over low heat and bring to a simmer. Then cover partially and reduce the liquid down to half its original volume (amount).
2. When it boils down to about a cup of liquid, strain out the herbs and add 8 ounces of honey.
3. Warm this mixture over low heat until well combined. Don't heat above 110 degrees.
4. Let cool completely before bottling.
5. Then pour syrup into bottles and label.
6. Store in the refrigerator up to six months.

Storage:
It should keep for a few weeks if refrigerated.

Recommended Dosage
The dose of the herbs depends on the type of herbs used.

TINCTURES

Tinctures are concentrated herbal extracts made by soaking the bark, berries, leaves (dried or fresh), or roots in alcohol or vinegar. The alcohol or vinegar pulls out the active ingredients in the plant parts, concentrating them as a liquid.

What issues are best addressed with tinctures?
Blood issues, Cough, asthma, arthritis, muscle spasms, sleep disorders, stomach issues, impotence, chronic skin diseases, injuries, and viral issues etc.

Best Part of the plant to use:

Bark, berries, leaves (dried or fresh), or roots from one or more plants in alcohol or vinegar.

Simple Recipe
- Fill up glass jar with herb halfway.
- Add vodka so that level of the liquid is at least two inches above the herb.
- Place parchment paper between the lid and jar.
- Seal jar tightly.
- Label jar with date, percentage alcohol, herbs, and method used.
- Shake two times per day for one month.

Supplies needed to prepare:
Glass jar
Dried Herbs
Vodka

Storage:
In general, the range you can expect your tincture to last is between six months and three years.

Recommended Dosage
The most commonly used dose for tinctures is 30-60 drops or 1-2 dropperfuls. In general, the more acute a condition, the more frequent the doses. Safe dosage ranges are fairly broad with most, but not all, herbs.

WASHES

Herbal washes are herb infusions that you use on the outside of the body.

Issues that can be addressed with herbal washes
Viral and bacterial eye infections and Skin Issues

Best part of the plant to use:
Flowers and leaves

Supplies needed to make herbal washes:
- 2 Tablespoons of herbs
- 2 cups distilled water
- 2 pinches of salt
- 2 glass eye cups
- Strainer or coffee filter

Simple Recipe:
- Steep the herbs in a covered pot for 15 to 20 minutes.
- Once finished, strain the herbs out of the tea through a strainer or thin filter to remove all the herb out of solution.
- Add the pinch of salt and stir until dissolved.
- After the liquid has cooled to room temperature, pour it in your eye cup to wash out your eyes.

Notice

With any of these methods, it's best to use distilled, filtered, or sterilized and boiled water to eliminate any opportunity for bacteria to get into the eye area.

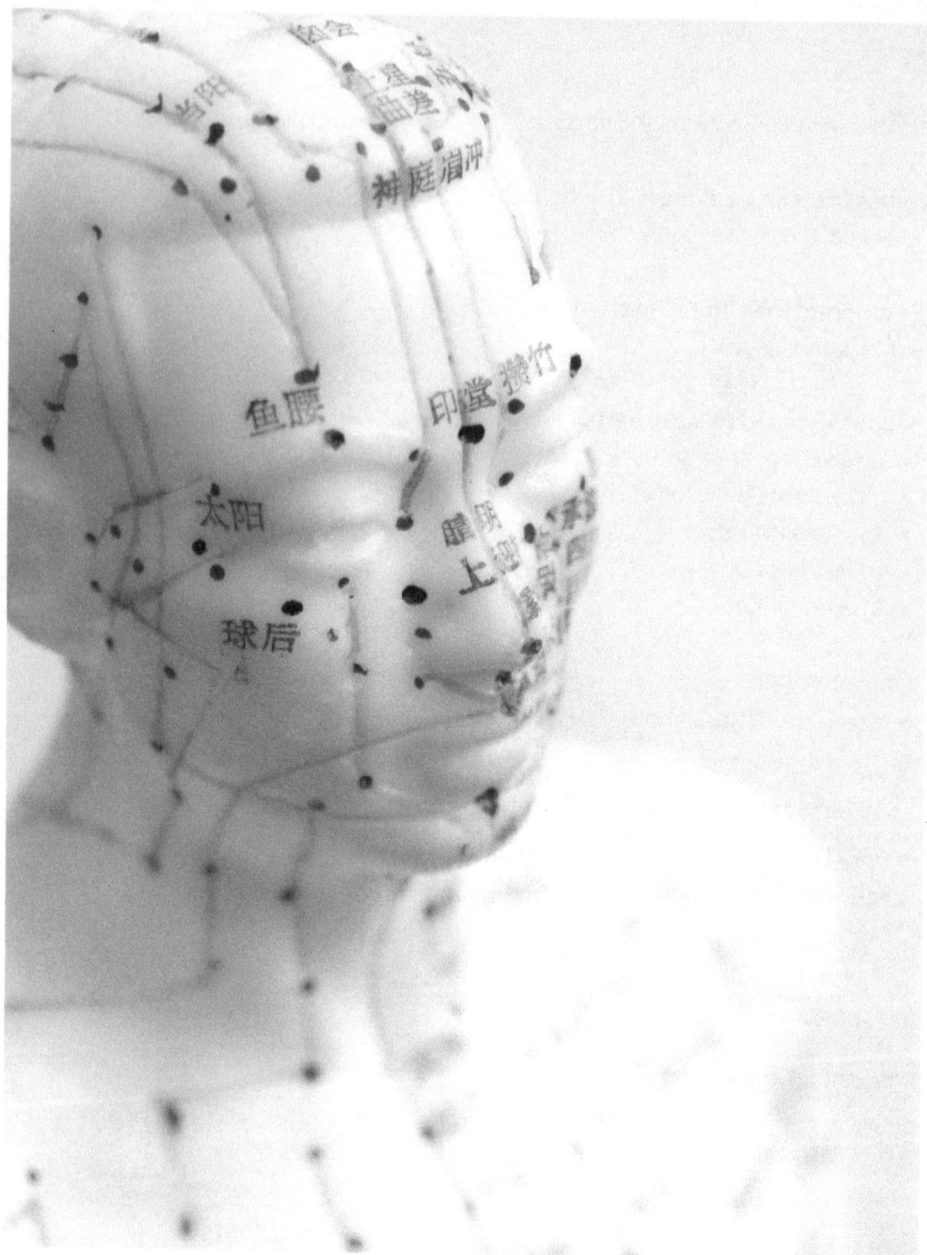

COMMON ISSUES

BACTERIAL INFECTION

Bacterial infections occur when bacteria enter the body, increase in number, and cause a reaction in the body.

Types

- Food poisoning (gastroenteritis).
- Some skin, ear or sinus infections.
- Some sexually transmitted infections (STIs).
- Bacterial pneumonia.
- Most urinary tract infections (UTIs).
- Strep throat
- Ear infections
- Pneumonia
- Bacterial vaginosis

Symptoms

- Fever
- Chills and sweats
- Swollen lymph nodes
- New or sudden worsening of pain
- Unexplained exhaustion
- Headache
- Skin flushing, swelling, or soreness
- Gastrointestinal symptoms, such as: nausea, vomiting, diarrhea, abdominal, or rectal pain.

Strategy

- Reduce toxic load
- Antiviral and Antibacterial herbs,
- Immune strengthening herbs, Febrifuge (reduce fever), Decongestant herbs (clear excess mucus)

Herbs

- Astragalus (Astragalus membr.)
- Boneset (Eupatorium perfolia.)
- Catnip (Nepeta cateria)
- Cayenne (Capsicum frutescens)
- Chamomile (Matricaria recutita)
- Echinacea (Echinacea angust.)
- Elderflower (Sambucus)
- Eucalyptus (Eucalyptus glob.)
- Garlic (Allium sativa)
- Ginger (Zingber officinale)
- Peppermint (Mentha piperita)
- Yarrow (Achillea millefolium)

Method of Administration

- Decoctions
- Douche
- Enemas
- Teas
- Tinctures

BITES AND STINGS

A bite is when an insect (like a mosquito, flea, or bedbug) uses its mouth to break a person's skin. A sting is a wound or pain caused by stinging.

Types

- Ant Bites
- Bug Bites
- Snake Bites
- Human/Animal Bites
- Bee and Wasp Stings

Symptoms

Bite

- Pain
- Swelling
- Redness
- Bleeding
- Swelling
- Itchy

Sting

- Pain
- Swelling
- Redness
- Itchiness
- Warmth
- Serious allergic reaction
- Coughing
- Tickling in throat

First Aid

Human/Animal Bite

1. Examine the wound. (Is the skin is broken

2. Wash the wound with antiseptic soap. Apply a bandage

3. If the skin is broken, see your doctor as soon as possible.

Snakebites

1. Make sure there is no danger of a second snakebite around.

2. Have the person sit down and keep the affected limb below the heart.

3. Flush the bite with soapy water.(do not apply cold compresses or ice).

4. Splint the limb as you would a broken bone.

5. Seek medical attention asap.

Stings

1. If you can see the insect's stinger, remove it as quickly as possible.

2. Wash the area with soap and water.

3. Apply ice wrapped in a towel or a cool wet cloth to the area to relieve pain and swelling.

Get Medical Care if:
- If you have a known severe allergy.
- Injectable epinephrine (EpiPen) was used
- Area shows signs of infection.

Herbs

- Aloe vera)
- Calendula (Calendula officinalis)
- Comfrey (Symphytum officinale)
- Plantain (Plantago)
- Witch hazel (Hamamelis)
- Yarrow (Achillea millefolium)

Method of Administration

- Compress
- Creams
- Salves

BLEEDING

Bleeding is the release of blood from a broken blood vessel, either inside or outside the body.

Types

- Wounds
- Nosebleed

Symptoms

External
- Confusion
- Clammy skin.
- Dizziness after an injury.
- Low blood pressure.
- Paleness
- Rapid pulse (increased heart rate)
- Shortness of breath.
- Weakness.

Internal
- Pain at the injury site.
- Swollen, tight abdomen.
- Nausea and vomiting.
- Pale, clammy, skin.
- Loss of breath.
- Extreme thirst.
- Unconscious

First Aid

Nosebleed

1. Pinch the entire soft part of the nose (above nostril)

2. Sit and lean forward

3. Breathe through your mouth.

4. Hold nose for 5 minutes. (add 10 min if nose keeps bleeding).

Wound

1. Examine the wound. (Is the skin is broken?)

2. NO, wash the wound with antiseptic soap. Apply a bandage.

3. YES, see your doctor as soon as possible.

Severe Bleeding

1. Remove any clothing or debris from the wound.

2. Stop the bleeding.

3. Lie the injured person down.

4. Add more bandages if needed.

Herbs

- Cypress (Cupressus sempervi.)
- Mugwort leaf (Artemisia vulg. L)
- Nettle (Urtica dioica)
- Shepherds purse (Capsella bu.)
- Turmeric (Curcuma longa)
- Uva Ursi (Arctostaphylos una u.)
- Yarrow (Achillea millefolium)

Methods of Administration

- Poultice
- Powder
- Tea

Caution
- Call 911 if the wound is deep or you're unsure of its seriousness.
- If nose bleed does not stop go to the emergency room.

BURNS

Before administering first aid for burns, you must be able to recognize the type of burn to be treated. Burns are tissue damage that occurs as a result of heat (fire, hot objects, hot liquids), chemical (wet or dry chemicals), or electrical (electrical wires, current, or lightning) contact. Burns are classified as first-, second-, or third-degree, depending on how deep and severe they penetrate the skin's surface.

Types

- Chemical
- Electrical
- Thermal

Symptoms

First-degree burns:
- Red skin
- Painful skin
- No blisters

Second-degree burns:
- Red skin
- Painful skin
- Blisters
- Swelling

Third-degree burns:
- White, black, deep red or charred skin
- Can be painful or numb

Fourth-degree burns:
- Lost feeling in area
- Skin tissue, fat, muscle and possibly bone destroyed

First Aid

Chemical
- Protect your eyes from chemical contamination.
- Remove dry chemicals. Put on gloves and brush off any remaining material.
- Remove contaminated clothing or jewelry and rinse chemicals off for at least 20 minutes.
- Bandage the burn.
- Rinse as needed.

Electrical
Major:
- Have someone call 911
- Do not touch the "electrified person" with your hands.
- Unplug the appliance or turn off the main power switch.
- Remove the person from the electrical source.
- Check to see if the person is responsive. If the person is not, start CPR.

Minor:
Rinse the burn with water, and apply a bandage.

Thermal
- Remove the person from the source of the burn.
- If the persons clothes are on fire, cover them with any large piece of nonsynthetic material
- Next, roll the person on the ground to put out the flames.

Herbs

- Aloe (Alore vera)
- Astragalus (Astragalus memb.)
- Calendula (Calendula officinal.)
- Comfrey (Symphytum offic.)
- Dragons blood (Croton lechleri)
- Tea tree oil (Melaleuca altern.)
- Witch hazel (Hamamelis virgin.)

Method of Administration
- Compress
- Poultice
- Tinctures

Caution
- Do not break blisters.
- Do not apply grease or ointments to the burns.
- Synthetic materials (i.e. nylon)may melt and cause further injury.

COLDS/FLU

The common cold is a viral infection of your nose and throat (upper respiratory tract). It is one of the bodys way of ridding itself of toxins, irritants, etc.The flu also known as, Influenza, is an infection of the nose, throat and lungs, which are part of your respiratory system.

Types

- Common Cold
- Rhinoviruses
- Parainfluenza
- Adenovirus
- Enterovirus
- Respiratory Syncytial Viruses

Symptoms

Common Cold

- Common Cold
- Sneezing
- Stuffy nose
- Runny nose
- Sore throat
- Coughin.
- Mucus dripping
- Watery eyes
- Fever

Flu

- Fever/chills.
- Cough.
- Sore throat.
- Runny or stuffy nose.
- Muscle or body aches.
- Headaches.
- Fatigue (tiredness)
- Vomiting
- Diarrhea

Strategy

Antiviral and Antibacterial herbs. Stimulate the immune system and build your resistance. Stay hydrated drinking, water, juice, clear broth or warm lemon water with honey to help loosen congestion and prevent dehydration.

Herbs

- Elder (Sambucus nigra)
- Garlic (Allium sativus)
- Ginger (Zingiber officinale)
- Ground Ivy (Glechoma hedera.)
- Lomatium (Lomatium dissec.)
- Peppermint (Mentha piperta)
- Siberian ginseng (Eleuthrococcus)
- St. johns wort (Hypericum per.)
- Wild indigo (Baptisia tinctoria)
- Yarrow (Achillea millefolium)

Method of Administration

- Decoctions
- Inhalations
- Teas
- Tinctures

DEHYDRATION

Dehydration is the absence of enough water in your body.

Types

- HYPOTONIC (LOSS OF ELECTROLYTES)

- HYPERTONIC (PRIMARILY LOSS OF WATER)

- ISOTONIC (EQUAL LOSS OF WATER AND ELECTROLYTES)

Symptoms

- Dizziness or light-headedness.
- Headache
- Tiredness
- Extreme thirst
- Dry mouth, lips and eyes
- Passing small amounts of urine infrequently

First Aid

- Take the person to a cool, shaded area.
- Encourage the person to sit down and stop any physical activity.
- Give plenty of water or Oral Rehydration Solution's (ORS) to drink
- If the person is suffering from cramps, stretch and massage the affected muscles.
- Monitor and record vital signs (eg: pulse / respiratory rate) if trained to do so.

Herbs

- Amla (Emblica officinalis)
- Asparagus (Asparagus offici.)
- Chamomile (Matricaria rec.)
- Cucumber ((Cucumis sati.)
- Tulsi (Ocimum basilicum)
- Willow Bark (Salix)

Method of Administration

- Drinks
- Teas

DIGESTIVE ISSUES

Gastroesophageal reflux disease (GERD) occurs when stomach acid frequently flows back into your esophagus.

Types

- Celiac Disease
- Crohn's Disease
- Irritable Bowel Syndrome (IBS)
- Ulcerative Colitis
- Upset stomach

Symptoms

- Bleeding
- Bloating and constipation
- Diarrhea
- Frequent discomfort
- Heartburn
- Nausea and vomiting
- Pain

Strategy

Eliminate toxins, soothe stomach irritation, eat easily digested foods until digestion is restored, address bleeding, and stop spasms and irritation.

Actions of herbs: Demulcents, Antibacterial, Vulneraries, Anti-inflammatory and Antispasmodic herbs.

Herbs

- Anise (Pimpinella anisum)
- Calamus (Acorus calamus)
- Cayenne (Capsicum fructe.)
- Comfrey (Symphytum offi.)
- Gentian (Gentiana lutea)
- Geranium (Pelargonium)
- Ginger (Zingiber officinale)
- Goldenseal (Hydrastis cand.)
- Licorice (Glycyrrhia glabra)
- Papaya (Carica papaya)
- Slippery elm (Ulmus rubra)

Method of Administration

- Herb Rolled Pills
- Infusions
- Teas
- Tinctures

EAR INFECTION

An ear infection (otitis media) is an infection of the middle ear.

Types

- Acute otitis media (AOM)
- Otitis media with effusion (OME)
- Otitis externa (swimmer's ear)

Symptoms

- Pain in the ear
- High temperature
- Being sick
- Yellow or green discharge
- Lack of energy
- Muffled hearing
- Discharge running out of the ear
- A feeling of pressure or fullness inside the ear
- Itching and irritation in the ear

Strategy

Balance intestinal microbe, remove food allergies, eliminate infection and toxins. Strengthen immune system, stop pain, and inflammation.

Herbs

- Astragalus (Astragalus L.)
- Echinacea (Exhinacea angust.)
- Garlic (Allium sativa)
- Goldenseal (Hydrastis canade.)
- Grapefruit seed extract (Citrus)
- Licorice (Glycyrrhiza glabra)
- Mullein (Vasbascum thapsus)
- Plantain (Plantago lanceolata)

Method of Administration

- Compress
- Infusions
- Infused Oils
- Teas
- Tinctures

EXTREME HEAT ILLNESS

Heat Illness is a condition resulting from the body's inability to cope with a particular heat load. Heatstroke treatment centers on cooling your body to a normal temperature to prevent or reduce damage to your brain and vital organs.

Types

- Heat Cramps
- Heat Exhaustion
- Heat Stroke
- Heat Syncope

Symptoms

- Confusion
- Altered mental status or slurred speech.
- Loss of consciousness (coma)
- Hot or dry skin
- Seizures
- Very high body temperature
- Lack of sweating
- Red, hot, and dry skin
- Muscle weakness or cramps
- Nausea and vomiting

First Aid

- Move person to a cool area and remove outer clothing
- Cool person with water, cold compresses, an ice bath, or fans
- Circulate air around the person to speed cooling
- Place cold, wet cloths or ice on head, neck, armpits, and groin
- Call emergency medical service if persons condition gets worse or they experience fainting, or confusion.

Herbs

- Chamomile (Matricaria rec.)
- Chrysanthemum (Chrysanthemum)
- Hibiscus (Hibiscus)
- Lavender (Lavandula)
- Lemon balm (Melissa officinalis)
- Lemongrass (Cymbopogon citrat.)
- Peppermint (Mentha piperita L)
- Spearmint (Mentha spicata)

Method of Administration

- Teas
- Tinctures

EXTREME COLD ILLNESS

Exposed to cold temperatures, your body begins to lose heat faster than it can be produced.

Types

- Chilblains
- Frostbite
- Hypothermia
- Trench Foot

Symptoms

- Shivering
- Exhaustion or feeling very tired
- Confusion
- Cold skin and a prickling feeling
- Numbness
- Red, white, bluish-white, grayish-yellow, purplish, brown or ashy, skin
- Hard or waxy-looking skin
- Fumbling hands
- Memory loss
- Slurred speech
- Drowsiness

Strategy

Hypothermia

1. CALL 9-1-1 or the local emergency number.
2. Gently move the person to a warm place.
3. Monitor breathing and circulation.
4. Give rescue breathing and CPR if needed.
5. Remove any wet clothing and dry the person off.
6. Warm the person slowly by wrapping them in blankets or by putting dry clothing on the person.

Frostbite

1. Move the person to a warm place.
2. Handle the area gently
3. Gently soak the affected area in warm. water until it is red and feels warm.
4. Loosely bandage the area with dry, sterile dressings.
5. If fingers or toes are frostbitten, place dry, sterile gauze between them.
6. Avoid breaking any blisters.
7. Do not allow the affected area to refreeze.
8. Seek professional medical care as soon as possible.

Herbs

- Cayenne (Capsicum fructes.)
- Cloves (Syzgium aromaticu.)
- Ginger (Zingiber officinale)
- Turmeric (Curcuma)

Method of Administration

- Decoctions
- Teas

EYE CONDITIONS

Disorders that impact the eye. The conjunctiva protects our eyes against many irritants(pollen, smoke, dust). When irritants get into the eye this can create issues of the eye.

Types

- Amblyopia
- Cataract
- Conjunctivitis (Pink Eye- inflammation)
- Diabetic Retinopathy
- Glaucoma
- Macular Degeneration
- Strabismus

Symptoms

- Red Eyes.
- Night Blindness
- Headache
- Light Sensitivity
- Floaters
- Flashes
- Dry Eyes
- Excessive Tearing
- Pink or red color in the white of the eye(s)
- Swelling of the conjunctiva and/or eyelids.
- Increased tear production.
- Itching, irritation, and/or burning

Strategy

Lubricate and soothe eyes. Decrease pressure in eyes. Eliminate toxins. Relieve pain. Address inflammation. Protect the structure of the eyes from free radical damage.

Actions of herbs: Antiseptic, Antimicrobial, Antioxidants, Anti-inflammatory, Anti-histimine .

Herbs

- Bilberry (Vaccinium myrtillus)
- Calendula (Calendula officinal.)
- Coleus (Coleus forskohili)
- Dusty miller (Cinerarea)
- Eyebright (Euphrasia officinalis)
- Goldenseal (Hydrastis canad.)
- Goldthread (Coptis trifolia)
- Grape seed extract (Vitis vinif.)
- Leutin (Spinach extract)

Method of Administration

- Compress
- Eye washes
- Tea bags
- Tinctures

FEVER

A fever is a temporary rise in body temperature.

Range

- Normal body temperature ranges from 97.5°F to 98.9°F (36.4°C to 37.2°C).

- It tends to be lower in the morning and higher in the evening.

- Most healthcare providers consider a fever to be 100.4°F (38°C) or higher.

Symptoms

High Grade (103°F (39.4°C) or above.):
- Sweating
- Chills and shivering
- Headache
- Muscle aches
- Loss of appetite
- Irritability
- Dehydration
- General weakness

Low Grade (between 100.4 and 102.2 degree):
- Warm skin
- A flushed face
- Glassy eyes
- Chills or Shivering
- Sweating
- Headache
- Muscle Aches

Strategy

Reduce or raise depending on the situation, eliminate toxins, drink plenty of fluids.

Herbs

- Catnip (Nepeta cataria)
- Echinacea (Echinacea angust.)
- Elderflowers (Sambucus)
- Lemon balm (Melissa officin.)
- Moringa (Moringa oleifera)
- White willow bark (Salix alba)
- Yarrow (Achillea millefolium)

Method of Administration

- Decoction
- Tea bags
- Tinctures

FIBROMYALGIA

Fibromyalgia is a chronic (long-lasting) disorder that causes pain and tenderness throughout the body.

Symptoms

- Fatigue
- Insomnia
- Fever
- Anxiety
- Pain and stiffness all over the body.
- Fatigue and tiredness.
- Depression and anxiety.
- Sleep problems.
- Problems with thinking, memory, and concentration.
- Headaches, including migraines.

Disorder linked to:

- Chronic fatigue syndrome
- Phosphorus deposits in the tissues
- Chemical sensitivities
- Chronic viral, bacterial, and parasitic infections.
- Irritable bowel syndrome (IBS)
- Depression
- Painful bladder syndrome

Strategy

This is a systemic condition that needs a multi-layered approach. Use herbs that address:
- Musculoskeletal System (muscles, joints, ligaments, etc.)
- Immune Modulators
- Hormone Modulators

Herbs

- Astragalus (Astragalus L)
- Black cohosh (Actaea racem.)
- Bosewelia (Boswellia sacra)
- Burdock (Arctium lappa)
- Cats claw (Uncaria tomentosa)
- Curcumin (Curcuma)
- Devils claw (Harpagophytum)
- Licorice (Glycyrrhiza glabra)
- Milk thistle (Silybum marian.)
- Olive leaf (Olea europaea)

Method of Administration

- Compress
- Decoctions
- Liniment
- Poultices
- Tinctures
- Topical

FRACTURES AND SPRAINS

A fracture is a break, usually in a bone. A sprain is a stretching or tearing of ligaments.

Types

Fracture:

- Greenstick
- Transverse
- Spiral
- Oblique

Sprain:

- Mild sprain: Little stretching of the ligaments.
- Moderate sprain: Combination of stretching and a little tearing of the ligament.
- Severe sprain: Complete tear of the ligament.

Symptoms

Fracture:

- A visibly out-of-place or mis-shapen limb or joint
- Swelling, bruising, or bleeding
- Intense pain
- Numbness and tingling
- Broken skin with bone sticking out
- Limited mobility

Sprain:

- Pain
- Swelling
- Bruising
- Limited mobility
- Hearing or feeling a "pop" in your joint at the time of injury.

First Aid

Sprain:
- **Rest** (Avoid activities that cause pain, swelling or discomfort)
- **Ice** (Ice the area immediately)
- **Compression** (Compress the area with an elastic bandage until the swelling stops)
- **Elevation** (Lift feet above the heart).

Fracture:
- Stop any bleeding.
- Apply pressure to the wound with a sterile bandage.
- Immobilize the injured area.
- Apply ice packs to limit swelling and help relieve pain.
- Treat for shock

Herbs

Fracture:
Cassia occidentalis (Fabaceae)
Cicuta maculata (Apiaceae)
Boneset (Eupatorium perfoliatum)

Sprain:
White willow (Salix alba)
Horse chestnut (Aesculus hippocastan).

Method of Administration

- Compress
- Decoction
- Tinctures
- Teas

FUNGAL INFECTIONS

Fungal infections, or mycosis, are dis-eases caused by a fungus (yeast or mold).

Types

- Aspergillosis
- Athlete's foot
- Blastomycosis
- Candidiasis
- Fungal Eye Infections
- Jock itch
- Onychomycosis
- Pityriasis versicolor
- Pneumonia
- Ringworm (dermatophytosis)
- Tinea versicolor
- Valley Fever
- Yeast infection

Symptoms

- Asthma-like symptoms
- Fatigue
- Headache
- Muscle aches or joint pain
- Night sweats
- Weight loss
- Chest pain
- Itchy or scaly skin
- Itching or vaginal discharge

Strategy

Reduce fungal growth and/or prevent infection. Address immune system and eliminate toxins.

Herb Actions:
Anti-fungal

Herbs

- Black walnut (Juglans nigra)
- Cats claw (Uncaria toment.)
- Garlic (Allium sativum)
- Goldenseal (Hydrastis can.)
- Grapefruit seed extract (Citrus)
- Neem (Azadirachta indica)
- Olive leaf (Olea europaea)
- Oregano oil (Origanum vulg.)
- Tea tree oil (Melaleuca alt.)

Method of Administration

- Creams
- Decoctions
- Douche
- Ointments
- Salves
- Suppositories
- Teas
- Tincture

HEADACHE

A painful sensation in any part of the head, ranging from sharp to dull, that could occur with other symptoms.

Types

- Tension Headache
- Sinus Headaches
- Exertion Headaches
- Migraines
- Hormone Headaches
- Cluster Headache
- Hypertension Headaches

Symptoms

- Slow onset of the headache.
- Head hurts on both sides.
- Dull pain or feels like a band or vice around the head.
- Pain in the back part of the head or neck.
- Pain is mild to moderate, but not severe.
- Vertigo
- Nausea
- Vomiting

Strategy

Address the liver, infection, toxicity, and digestive and respiratory issues.

Herb Actions:
Anti-inflammatory, Anti-spasmodic, Anti-nausea, Pain Relieving

Herbs

- Betony (Betonica officinalis)
- Chamomile (Matricaria recutita)
- Dandelion (Taraxacum)
- Kava kava (Piper methysticum)
- Lavender (Lavandula)
- Milk thistle (Silybum marianum)
- Petasites (Petasites japonicus)
- Valerian (Valeriana officinalis)
- Verbena (Verbena)
- White Willow Bark (Salix alba)

Method of Administration

- Compress
- Teas
- Tinctures

HEART ISSUES

Heart conditions that affects your vessels, structural problems, and blood clots.

Types

- Heart attack
- Heart failure
- Arrhythmias
- Valve disease
- High blood pressure
- Congenital heart conditions

Symptoms

- Chest pain or discomfort
- Shortness of breath
- Pain or discomfort in the jaw, neck, back, arm, or shoulder
- Feeling nauseous
- Light-headed.
- Chest tightness
- Chest pressure and chest discomfort (angina)
- Indigestion
- Heartburn
- Nausea
- Swelling in your legs

First Aid

How to treat a Stroke:
- Call 9-1-1
- Make sure the person is in a safe and comfortable position.
- Check to see if the person is breathing.
- If not, start CPR. If they are having trouble breathing, loosen any tight clothing.
- Cover them with a blanket to keep them warm.
- Do not give food or water.
- Observe their condition until medical help arrives.

How to treat a Heart Attack:
- Call 9-1-1.
- Sit or lie the person down and loosen any clothing.
- Monitor symptoms and pulse.
- Begin CPR if the casualty goes unconscious and isn't breathing.

Herbs

Bromelain (Ananas comosus)
Coleus (Coleus forskolii)
Curcumin (Turmeric)
Dong quai (Angelica sinensis)
Ginko (Ginko biloba)
Green tea (Camellia Sinensis)
Hawthorn (Crataegus oxycantha)
Red sage (Saliva miltiorrhiza)

Arjuna (Terminalia arjuna)
Butchers broom (Ruscus aculeatus)
Garlic (Allium sativa)
Horse chestnut (Aeschlus hippocas.)
Motherwort (Leonarus cardiaca)
Shepherds purse (Capsella bursa past.)
Valerian (Valeriana officinalis)
Yarrow (Achilla millefolium)

INFLAMMATION

Inflammation is part of the body's defense mechanism. It is the process by which the immune system recognizes and removes harmful and foreign stimuli and begins the healing process.

Types

Acute inflammation:
- The response to sudden body damage, such as stabbing your leg.

Chronic inflammation:
- Your body continues sending inflammatory cells even when there is no outside danger. Long term inflammation lasting months to years.

Symptoms

- Fever
- Chills
- Fatigue/loss of energy
- Headaches
- Loss of appetite
- Muscle stiffness

Strategy

Clear toxins, reduce pro-inflammation substances, address stress, supply nutrient deficiencies, clean and strengthen liver.

Herb Actions:
Anti-inflammatory, Pain Reliever, Tissue Repair

Herbs

- Boswellia (Boswellia sacra)
- Chamomile (Matricaria re.)
- Flaxseed (Linum usitatiss.)
- Ginger (Zingiber officinale)
- Hawthorn (Crataegus oxyc.)
- Licorice (Glycyrrhiza glabra)
- Meadowsweet (Filipeandu.)
- Quercetin (Quercus)
- Willow bark (Salix spp.)
- Yarrow (Achilla millefolium)

Method of Administration

- Decoctions
- Salves
- Teas
- Tinctures
- Poultices

NAUSEA

A feeling of sickness with an inclination to vomit.

Common Causes

- Medication
- Gallbladder disease
- Food poisoning
- Heart attack
- Concussion
- Brain tumor
- Ulcers
- Gastroparesis
- Pain
- Headache
- Anxiety/Stress
- Parasites
- Food allergies

Symptoms

- Feeling like you are about to vomit.
- Lack of appetite
- Profuse sweating
- Repeated rhythmic contractions of respiratory and abdominal muscles
- Stomachache
- Uneasy feeling in your chest
- Vomiting

Strategy

Hydrate, relieve stomach irritation, cleanse toxins, counter chronic infection, improve digestion, monitor food allergies, and emotional stress.

Herb Actions:
Analogous herbs, Anti-nausea herbs

Herbs

- Cayenne (Capsicum frutes)
- Cinnamon (Cinnamomum ze.)
- Cloves (Eugenia caryophyll.)
- Fennel (Foeniculum vulgare)
- Ginger (Zingiber officinale)
- Marshmallow (Althea officin.)
- Meadowsweet (Filipendula u.)
- Patchouli (Pogostemon cab.)
- Peppermint (Mentha piperta)
- Raspberry leaf (Rubus idaeus)

Method of Administration

- Decoctions
- Herb rolled pills
- Medicinal wines
- Tinctures

PARASITES

A parasite is an organism that lives on or in a host and gets its food at the expense of its host.

Types

- Fascioliasis (Fasciola Infection)
- Filariasis (Lymphatic Filariasis, Elephantiasis)
- Foodborne Diseases
- Giardiasis (Giardia Infection)
- Gnathostomiasis (Gnathostoma Infection)
- Guinea Worm Disease (Dracunculiasis)
- Head Lice Infestation

Symptoms

- Abdominal pain
- Diarrhea
- Nausea or vomiting
- Gas or bloating
- Dysentery (loose stools containing blood and mucus)
- Rash or itching around the rectum or vulva
- Stomach pain or tenderness
- Feeling tired

Strategy

Get rid of parasites, their larvae, and eggs.

Herb Actions:
Anti-parasitic herbs, remove toxins, parasite cleanse,

Herbs

- Cloves (Eugenia caryophylla.)
- Fennel (Foeniculum vulgare)
- Garlic (Allium sativa)
- Green black walnut hull (Juglans.)
- Pumpkin seeds (Curcubita p.)
- Wormwood (Artemisia absinthi.)

Method of Administration

- Ointments
- Salves
- Teas
- Tinctures

POISON

A poison is defined as a substance that can cause harm to the body when consumed or inhaled

Types

- Pesticides
- Carbon Monoxide
- Household products
- Inhalants
- Mercury Poison
- Botulinum Toxin
- Pharmaceuticals
- Organic solvents
- Drugs of abuse
- Industrial chemicals

Symptoms

- Headaches
- Nausea
- Vomiting
- Dizziness
- Irritation of the skins, eyes and mucous membranes.

Strategy

- Call poison control if you ingested poison
- Remove poison and toxins from system.

Herb Actions:
Emetic Herbs

Herbs

- Activated black charcoal
- Bayberry (Myrica cerifera)
- Blessed Thistle (Cnicus ben.)
- Bloodroot (Sanguinaria cana.)
- Chaparral (Larrea tridentata)
- Vervain (Verbena)
- Yucca (Yucca ssp.)

Method of Administration

- Decoction
- Tincture

SHOCK

Shock is a critical condition brought on by the sudden drop in blood flow through the body. When a person is in shock, his or her organs aren't getting enough blood or oxygen.

Causes

- Trauma
- Heatstroke
- Blood loss
- An allergic reaction
- Severe infection
- Poisoning
- Severe burns
- Malfunctioning heart

Symptoms

- Cool, clammy skin
- Pale or ashen skin
- Bluish tinge to lips or fingernails (or gray in the case of dark complexions)
- Rapid pulse
- Rapid breathing
- Nausea or vomiting
- Enlarged pupils
- Weakness or fatigue

First Aid

- Don't not allow the person to move. Lie the person down and raise the legs to encourage more blood flow to the heart, lungs, and head until medical help comes.
- **Begin CPR if the person shows no signs of life, such as not breathing or moving.**
- Loosen tight clothing
- Cover the person with a blanket to prevent chilling (if needed).
- Don't let the person eat or drink anything.

First Aid for Shock

- Call 911
- Lay the Person Down, if Possible.
- Begin CPR, if Necessary.
- Treat Obvious Injuries.
- Keep Person Warm and Comfortable.
- Follow Up

Helpful Herbs

Shock brought on by physical trauma:
Cayenne (Capsicum fructescens)
Arnica (Arnica montana)

Shock brought on by emotional trauma:
Skullcap (Scutellaria lateriflora)
Valerian (Valeriana officinalis)
Arnica (Arnica montana)
Cherry Plum (Prunus cerasifera)

SKIN ISSUES

Disorders or issues with the skin.

Types

- Eczema
- Psoriasis
- Acne
- Rosacea
- Ichthyosis
- Vitiligo
- Hives.
- Seborrheic dermatitis

Symptoms

- Discolored skin patches
- Dry skin
- Flushed skin
- Open sores, lesions or ulcers
- Peeling skin
- Rashes, possibly with itchiness or pain
- Red, white or pus-filled bumps
- Scaly or rough skin
- Dark spots

Strategy

Address liver and colon toxins, detoxify blood, boost immune system, and remove allergens.

Herb Actions:
Antiseptics, Astringents, Emollients, Rubefacients, Styptics, Vulneraries

Herbs

- Aloe (Aloe vera)
- Bitter melon (Momordica ch.)
- Burdock (Articum lappa)
- Calendula (Calendula offic.)
- Cardiospermum (Cardiosper.)
- Chickweed (Stellaria media)
- Evening primrose (Oenether.)
- Heal-all (Prunella vulgaris)
- Horse chestnut (Aesculus h.)
- Licorice (Glycyrrhiza glabra)
- Plantain (Plantago lance.)
- Witch hazel (Hamamelis vir.)

Method of Administration

- Compress
- Creams
- Hand rolled pills
- Ointment
- Teas
- Tinctures

TOOTH ISSUES

Issues with your teeth.

Types

- Gum Disease
- Tooth Sensitivity
- Tooth Decay
- Oral Cancer
- Dry Mouth

Symptoms

- Toothache
- Tooth sensitivity
- Grey, brown or black spots appearing on your teeth.
- Bad breath

Strategy

Healthy diet, fight infection, remove toxins, stop decay, pain relief.

Herbs

- Cloves (Syzygium aromat.)
- Garlic (Allium sativum)
- Green tea (Camellia sinen.)
- Hydrogen peroxide (food grade)
- Licorice root (Glycyrrhiza.)
- Neem bark (Azadirachta i.)
- Oil of oregano (Origanum v.)
- Saltwater
- Turmeric (Curcuma)

Method of Administration

- Compress
- Gargles
- Tinctures
- Teas
- Washes

URINARY SYSTEM ISSUES

Issues that affect your urinary tract.

Types

- Urinary tract infections
- Kidney stones
- Kidney failure
- Interstitial cystitis
- Bladder control problems
- Prostate problems

Symptoms

- A strong urge to urinate that doesn't go away.
- A burning feeling when urinating.
- Urinating often, and passing small amounts of urine.
- Urine that looks cloudy.
- Urine that appears red or bright pink.
- Strong-smelling urine.

Strategy

Clear infections and inflammation, increase the flow of urine, heal and protect tissue linings, and regenerate kidney tissue.

Herbal Actions:
Diuretics, Antiseptic, Antilithics, Kidney tonics, Antibacterial, Anti-fungal

Herbs

- Buchu (Barosma betulina)
- Corn silk (Zea mays)
- Dandelion (Taraxacum officina)
- Goldenrod (Solidago virgaurea)
- Gravel root (Eupatorium pur.)
- Horsetail (Equisetum arvense)
- Hydrangea (Hydrangea arbo.)
- Juniper (Juniperus communis)
- Parsley root (Petroselinum cri.)

Method of Administration

- Decoctions
- Herbal Wines
- Teas
- Tinctures

VIRUSES

A virus is an infectious microbe consisting of a segment of nucleic acid (either DNA or RNA) surrounded by a protein coat.

Types

- Influenza (the flu)
- HIV, which can lead to AIDS
- Meningitis
- Pneumonia
- Human papillomavirus (HPV)
- Herpes
- Rotavirus

Symptoms

- Fever
- Head and body aches
- Fatigue
- Sore throat
- Cough
- Sneezing
- Nausea
- Vomiting
- Diarrhea
- Rashes
- Sores,
- Blisters
- Warts

Strategy

Remove toxins and address viral infections.

Herb Actions:
Antivirals, Anti-fungals

Herbs

- Astragalus Root (Astragalus)
- Cat's Claw (Uncaria toment.)
- Cranberry (Vaccinium macro.)
- Elderberry (Sambucus nigra)
- Garlic (Allium sativa)
- Ginger (Zingiber officinale)
- Lemon balm (Melissa officinal)
- Oregano oil (Origanum vulga)
- Turmeric (Curcuma)

Method of Administration

- Decoctions
- Inhalations
- Teas
- Tinctures

WOUNDS AND BRUISES

It is a basic term that refers to harm or damage to your body caused by falls, accidents, weapons, and hits.

Types

- Cuts
- scratches
- bruises
- lacerations
- Penetrating wounds
- Puncture wounds
- Surgical wounds and incisions
- Thermal, chemical or electric burns
- Bites and stings
- Gunshot wounds
- Blunt force trauma
- Abrasions
- Lacerations
- Skin tears

Symptoms

- Bleeding or oozing of blood
- Redness
- Swelling
- Pain and tenderness
- Heat
- Possible fever with infection.
- Poor movement of affected area.
- Oozing pus, foul smell

First Aid for Wounds/Bruises

- Wash your hands. This helps avoid infection.
- Stop the bleeding. Apply gentle pressure, if needed, with a clean bandage or cloth and elevate the wound to stop bleeding.
- Clean the wound. Rinse the wound with water. Wash around the wound with soap. Don't get soap in the wound.
- Remove any dirt or debris with a tweezers cleaned with alcohol.
- Apply a thin layer of an antibiotic ointment to keep the surface moist and help prevent scarring.
- Cover the wound. Apply a bandage, rolled gauze or gauze held in place with paper tape.
- Watch for signs of infection. See a doctor if you see signs of infection on the skin or near the wound, such as redness, increasing pain, drainage, warmth or swelling.

Herbs

- Aloe (Aloe vera)
- Calendula (Calendula officinalis)
- Tea tree oil (Melaleuca alternifolia)
- Marshmallow (Althea officinalis)
- Dragons blood (Croton lechleri)

Method of Administration

- Compresses
- Creams
- Ointments
- Tinctures
- Topicals

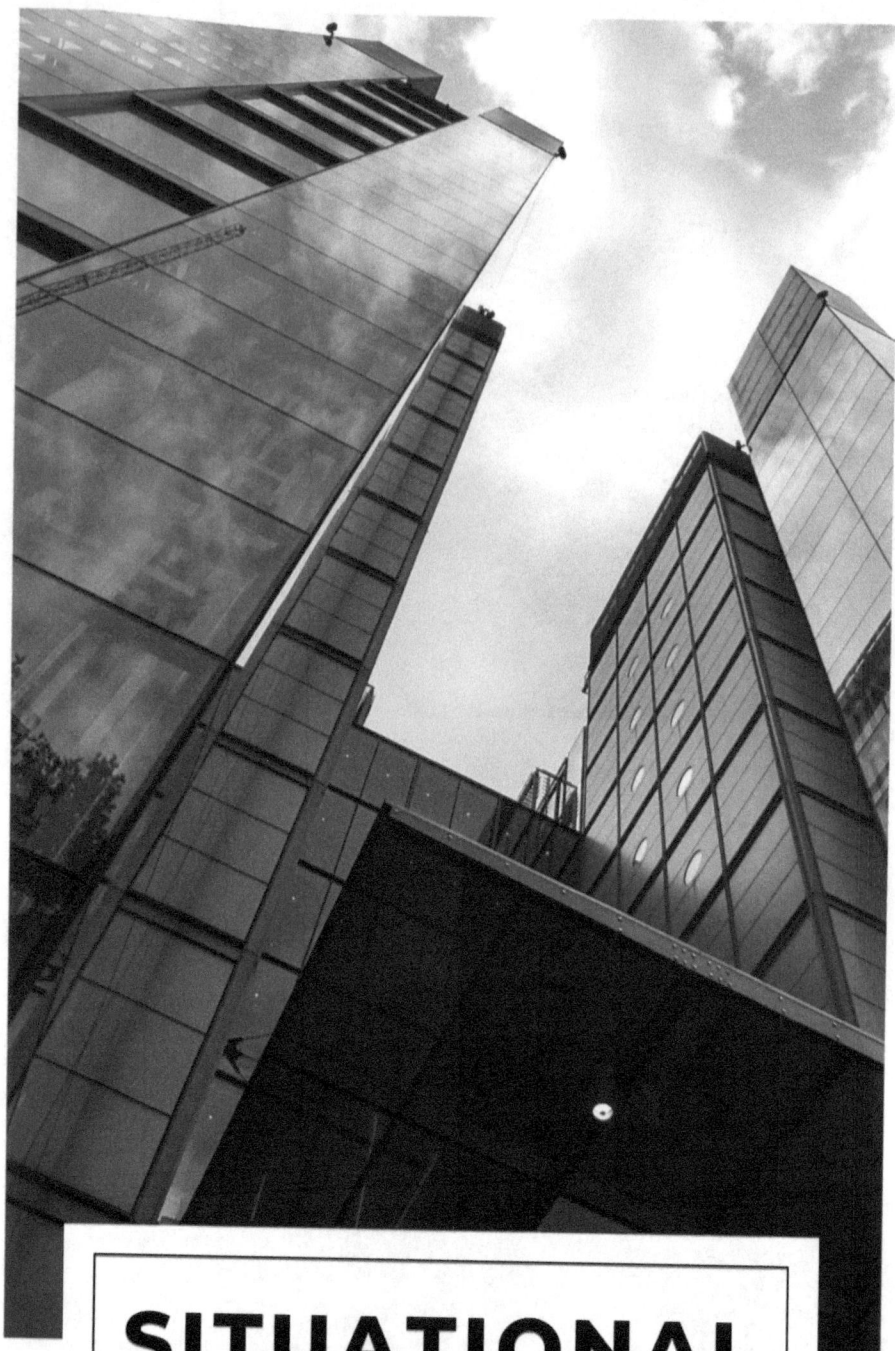

SITUATIONAL

FIRST AID

Urban Survival

Urban survival is the ability to survive an extended disaster in a city by using the necessary skills and tactics.

Urban survival is defined as having the skills and abilities to survive a crisis in a city. This goes beyond power outages and lock downs. This reaches far into other issues that people are dealing with on a daily basis such as job loss, crime, food shortages etc. Having the right skills to be able to survive in the city are just as important as being out in the wild. Sure the risks are different, however there are still risks and our body has no way to know is you are suffering from stress due to job loss or if there is a lion chasing you in the wild. It prepares the body the same way once that stress switch is turned on.

Some argue that it would be more difficult to survive in an urban area than a wilderness. They state that if a crisis or an emergency occurs, and there are various threats coming at you from all over, every person in the city would fight to gain valuable resources, so you won't be fighting alone there. This is true whether its as extreme as a riot or as mild as someone getting the job over you. The urban environment has its own issues that you have to be prepared for. Some of the following issues you might come in contact with in an urban setting are:

Food shortages/deserts
Job loss
Medication shortage
Poor water quality
Poverty

POOR AIR (POLLUTION)

Pollution is the placing of harmful materials into the environment. Air pollution is caused by solid and liquid particles and certain gases that are placed in the air. Pollution can come from factories, dust, pollen, car and truck exhaust, mold spores, wildfires and in some areas ,volcanoes.

Effects on our health:

Poor air quality can have many negative effects on our health. They can irritate our eyes, nose and throat, cause shortness of breath, irritate asthma and other respiratory issues, and impact the heart and cardiovascular system. Breathing polluted air for long periods of time can cause more serious problems such as cancer (lung), stokes, heart disease and chronic obstructive pulmonary disease (COPD).

Strategy
Detoxify and purify body and lungs

Herbs

Turmeric (Curcuma longa)- Turmeric helps ward off the toxic effects of inhaling polluted air

Neem (Azadirachta indica)- Neem can help absorb pollutants and detoxify the the body.

Giniger (Zingiber officinale)- The active compounds in ginger help combat nausea and cold as a result of pollution exposure.

Bhumiamla (Phyllanthus niruri)-This herb helps to purify blood and get rid of the waste materials from the body.

Amlaki (Emblica officinalis)-Detoxifies the body from harmful chemicals.

Tulsi (Ocimum tenuiflorum)-Herb used for protection and detoxification.

Ghrit Kumari (Aloe barbadensis). Succulent herb that has the property to clean organic by-products such as formaldehyde and benzene .

POOR WATER QUALITY

Water is essential to human life. It is stated that "Of six environmental problems facing the U.S., Americans remain most worried about those that affect water quality. Majorities express "a great deal" of worry about the pollution of both drinking water (56%) and rivers, lakes and reservoirs (53%)(1)."All across the United States people are being exposed to and drinking unsafe water. Pollutants such as metals, oils, pesticides, and fertilizers run off from land into the waters, causing several damaging impacts.

Effects on our health

Exposure to high doses of chemicals can lead to health issues such as, skin discoloration, nervous system or organ damage, developmental or reproductive effects,and waterborne diseases caused by microbes (such as typhoid fever or cholera). The more common illnesses caused by viruses, bacteria, and parasites can result in diarrhea, fever, vomiting, headache, kidney failure, and stomach pain.

Water Purification Herbs:

Tamarai Nelumbium (Nelumbo nucifera)- Placed in wells, ponds and in biowastes to cleanse all impurities in water and to remove bad odors.

Cilantro (Coriandrum sativum)- The herb uses bio-absorption processes to remove toxins from water.

Daisy plant (Tridax procumbens)- This plant has the ability to remove fluoride and other heavy metals from drinking water through bio-absorption processes.

Moringa (Moringa oleifera)- Studies show that moringa seed powder is a natural coagulant and flocculent to clarify turbid water and copper as an antibacterial agent to destroy pathogens like E. coli to produce clean drinking water (2).

Water Purification Tools/Methods

- Boil your water- If you're at an elevation over 6,500 feet, bring the water to a rolling boil for 3 minutes.
- Sawyer Squeeze- Removes 99.99% of bacteria.
- Water purification tablets- Contain iodine, which kills bacteria and viruses.
- Activated charcoal water filters- Purifies water, balances pH, and removes contaminates.

1. Water Pollution Remains Top Environmental Concern in U.S. Brenan
https://news.gallup.com/poll/347735/water-pollution-remains-top-environmental-concern.aspx
2. Birnin-Yauri, U.. (2012). The use of some plants in water purification. 1. 71-75.

POVERTY

Poverty is about not having enough money to meet basic needs including food, clothing and shelter. Its been said that over 648 million people in the world, about eight percent of the global population, live in extreme poverty, which means they subsist on less than US$2.15 per day (1). According to the US Census, 37.9 million people are in poverty. what is the most important but what is often ignored consciously or unconsciously is how the urban poverty population with limited resources and property maintain their life. The urban poor living a life of uncertainty and insecurity throughout the year, are compelled to adopt various survival strategies to meet the challenges of their daily existence. Most people when they think about poverty immediately think about homelessness. who have a roof over their heads and a place to call home but may still be struggling to make ends meet

Effects on our health?

Poverty can cause mental illness, chronic disease, higher mortality, and lower life expectancy. Poverty also puts people at risk for chronic conditions such as heart disease, anxiety, diabetes and obesity.

Survival Strategy

- Set a crisis budget, prioritize bills and debts.
- Establish a family or community network.
- Consider alternative ways to make additional income.
- Change your consumption pattern.
- Reduce non-food resources
- Reduce stressors on body
- Address stress related illnesses
- Keep a positive mentality

Remedy

Resilience
Self-sufficiency
Creative thinking
Determination

Herbs that support a stressed body : Ashwaghanda(Withania somnifera), Valerian root(Valeriana officinalis)

1. Half of the global population lives on less than US$6.85 per person per day
https://blogs.worldbank.org/developmenttalk/half-global-population-lives-less-us685-person-day.

JOB LOSS

Being employed and being able to support yourself and your family provides a strong sense of control, builds confidence, and self esteem. However when someone loses their job that can challenge their sense of control. Job loss impacts the person first mentally and then over time it manifests physically.

Effects on our health?

Those who have lost their job have reported feelings of depression, anxiety, low self-esteem, and worry. On a physical level unemployed people have experienced stress-related illnesses such as high blood pressure, stroke, heart attack, heart disease, and arthritis.

Strategy

- Accept any frustration and anger that might have occurred as a result of your job loss. Don't suppress those feelings. Feel them and move forward.
- Decide if you want to go look for a job or use your gifts and talents to work for yourself
- Determine what your household bills are and set a plan to see how much income you need coming in. budget
- Set a plan and get to action
- Lean on your support system.
- Assess situation.
- Determine strengths and weaknesses.
- Decide to do something about it.

FOOD SHORTAGES/DESERTS

A shortage of food may happen when not enough food is produced, such as when crops fail due to drought, pests, or too much moisture.

Effects on our health?

Food insecurity and the lack of access to affordable nutritious food are associated with increased risk for multiple chronic health conditions such as diabetes , obesity, heart disease, mental health disorders and other chronic diseases. Continuous production of high yield GMO crops to supplement food shortages negatively impact our health.

How to survive a Food Shortage

- Don't panic buy, Meal Plan
- Know what wild game and fish are in your area
- Eat less meat
- Learn what edible fruits and plants grow around you
- Purchase foods that stretch (rice, beans, flour etc.) and can goods.
- Know how to filter water
- Know where local pantry's are in your area.
- If possible, start growing your own food.
- During times when food is in abundance prepare for times when it is not.

Common Edible Plants:

- Pine Nuts (Pinus Pinea)
- Chickweed (Stellaria media)
- Dandelion (Taraxacum officinale)
- Black Raspberries (Rubus occident.)
- Amaranth (Amaranthus retroflexus
- Asparagus (Asparagus officinalis)
- Burdock (Arctium lappa)
- Chicory (Cichorium intybus)
- Green Seaweed (Ulva lactuca)
- Kelp (Alaria esculenta)
- Plantain (Plantago)
- Prickly Pear Cactus (Opuntia)
- Wild Blackberries (Rubus ulmifo.)
- Dock (Rumex crispus)
- Grape Leaves (Vitis species)
- Miner's Lettuce (Claytonia perfol.)
- Nettle (Urtica dioica)
- Watercress (Nasturtium offici.)

Keep In Mind

- Be cautious. Make sure you can identify a plant with 100 percent certainty before touching or consuming it.
- Get a good field manual to help you identify what is growing in your area.
- Don't take more food than you need.
- Be aware of poisonous plant look-a-likes.

SURVIVE

MEDICATION SHORTAGE

The Federal Food, Drug, and Cosmetic Act defines a drug shortage as a period of time when the demand or projected demand for the drug within the United States exceeds the supply of the drug.

Effects on our health?

The direct impact renders patients unable to prevent and treat their diseases.

Strategy

Use herbal remedies to address common ailments.
Know what is growing in your area and what has medicinal value.
Take classes on how to make herbal remedies to address your ailments.
Seek the advice of an herbalist.

Herbs for pain
- White Willow Bark (Salix alba)
- White Oak Bark (Quercus)
- Jamaican Dogwood (Piscidia pi.)
- Aspen or Cottonwood buds
- Black Cohosh (Actea racemosa)

Anti-histamine herbs
- White Oak (Quercus alba)
- Grindelia (Grindelia lanceolat)
- Goldenrod (Solidago)
- Nettles (Urtica dioica)
- Fireweed (Chamaenerion angus.)
- Chickweed (Stellaria media)
- Plantain (Plantago)

Antibiotics
- Oil of Oregano (Origanum vulga.)
- Garlic (Allium sativum)

Nausea
- Cloves (Syzygium aromaticum)
- Ginger (Zingiber officinale)
- Fennel (Foeniculum vulgare)
- Peppermint (Mentha piperita L)
- Raspberry Leaf (Rubus idaeus)

Dental Care Herbs
- Clove (Cloves (Syzygium aroma.)
- Myrrh (Commiphora myrrha)
- Oregon Grape Root (Berberis aq.)
- White Oak (Quercus alba)
- Propolis (Apis mellifera)
- Peppermint (Mentha piperita L)

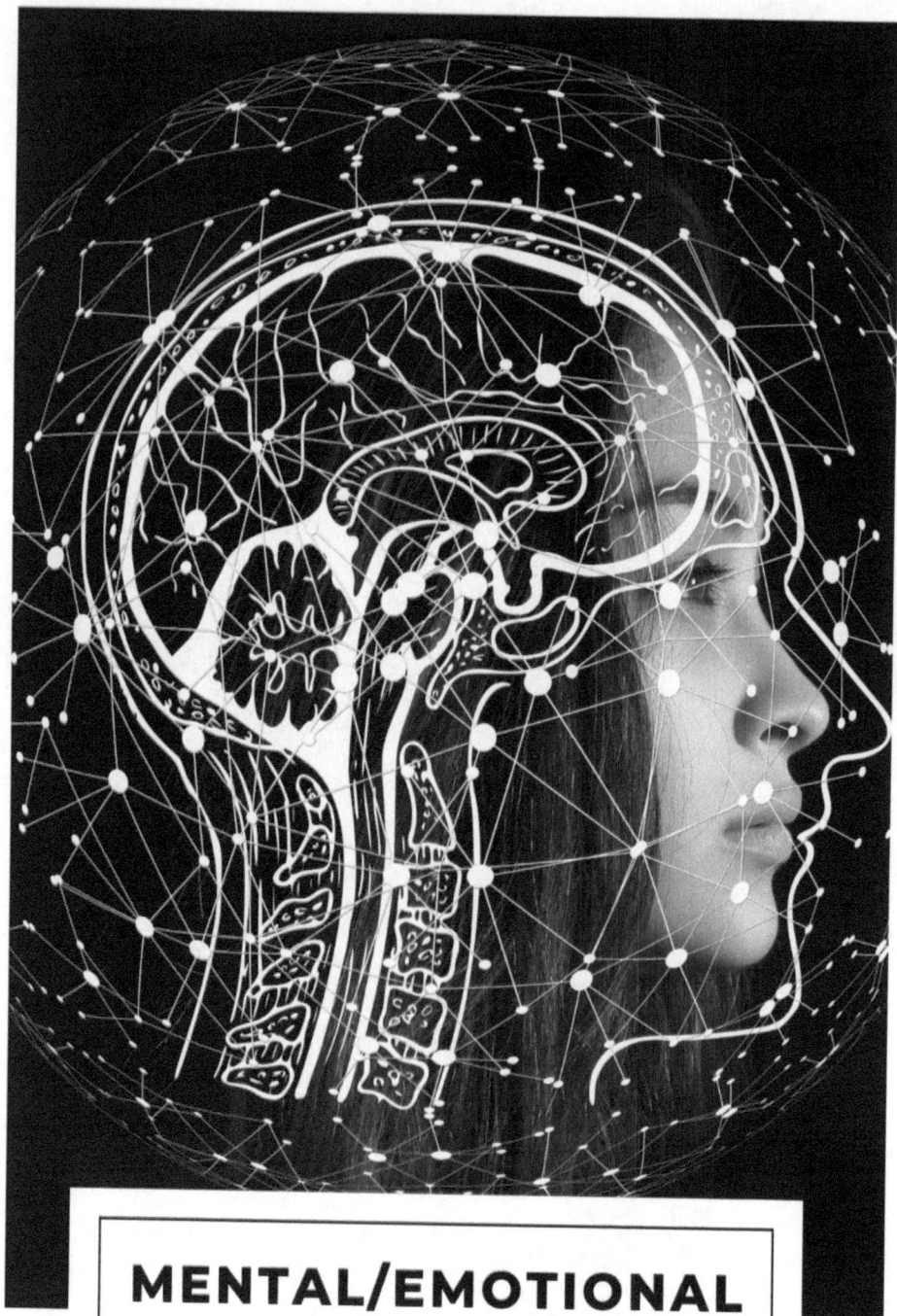

MENTAL/EMOTIONAL

FIRST AID

SKILLS NEEDED TO MANAGE PSYCHOLOGICAL ISSUES

This section is just as important as the others because it is important to understand how to handle the psychological issues that come our way. There is a link between the mind and the body and what you deal with emotionally can manifest physically into dis-ease or dis-order in the body. There is a lot of research on the mind and body connection and researchers have discovered several emotions that are linked to issues such as heart disease, cancer, hypertension, and immune disorders. As the date of this book the Centers for Disease Control (CDC) reports that 6 out of 10 adults have a chronic disease and 4 out of 10 have more than one chronic disease(1). The CDC also reported that 58.5 million Americans have arthritis and cancer is the second leading cause of death in the United States. Mental health disorders are also on the rise. According to the National Institutes of Health (NIH), nearly 1 in every 5 American adults live with an mental illness. The CDC reported that poor mental health amongst children is a huge concern. They stated that ADHD and anxiety plague 1 out of every 11 children.

What does all this mean?

This means we are in trouble. This means that people are struggling mentally and emotionally. This means that people are lacking the skills to be able to handle the stresses of life. It says that there is a gap in the knowledge of how to handle stress, trauma, and pressure. Today we live in a pressure cooker. Our society is highly self-centered, have it all right now, hyper-stimulated, and overly burdened. Long gone are the days of focusing on faith, family, and love. The above statistics show that we have lost our way and because of this we have paid a heavy price. We traded community, forgiveness, knowledge of self, spirituality, respect of each other and our lands, for selfishness, rage, convenience, greed, manipulation, worry, fear, resentment, disappointment, anger, bitterness, and unforgiveness. These negative characteristics is writing a check that our body has to cash. We can try to deny it all we want but guess what....our body keeps the score. I will say it again. Whatever you are dealing with mentally, if not addressed will manifest physically.

So whats the solution? **Change.** Don't wait until the doctor has told you that you have 6 months to live to start focusing on what is truly important and address the root issues. Education is key. Arming yourself with the characteristics needed to handle the trials of life is vital. You need to arm yourself with the following characteristics:

Spirituality (prayer)	Strength	Determination
Courage	Wisdom	Perseverance
Ability to adapt and adjust	Resilience	Empathy
Creativity	Good health	Discipline

PSYCHOLOGICAL FIST AID (PFA)

Psychological First Aid (PFA) is defined as a set of skills and knowledge that can be used to help people who are in distress. It is a way of helping people to feel calm and able to cope in a difficult situation. It is assisting people with emotional distress whether it results from physical injury, natural disaster, job loss. divorce, disease, death, grief, unmet expectations, trauma, or excessive stress/fear/anger. They could be dealing with over excitement, severe fear, excessive worry, deep depression, misdirected irritability, and anger and have reached the point of interfering with effective coping.

Some common symptoms that people might need PFA:

- Becomes socially withdrawn
- Symptoms of anxiety
- Depression
- Substance abuse
- Confusion
- Fear
- Feelings of hopelessness and helplessness
- Physical pain
- Anxiety
- Anger
- Grief
- Loss of appetite
- Headaches or chest pain
- Nausea, stomach pain
- Diarrhea
- Hyperactivity
- Sleep issues

Steps to Psychological First Aid

Psychological first aid is calming, emotional support, active listening and practical assistance. It is not counseling or treatment. It focuses on providing emotional and practical support. You can accomplish this in three easy steps, look, listen and link.

Look	Listen	Link
• Who needs help • Safety and Security risks • physical injury • immediate basic needs	• Actively listen • Accepts persons feelings • Calms the person • Helps find solution to immediate problems	• Connect with support systems • Tackle practical problems • Access information

Keep in mind:
- Life is cyclical. No experience is ever permanent. This too shall pass.
- Refer people for more specialized help if there is a medical issue or deeper psychological issue (self-harm, suicide attempt, prolonged grief, panic attacks, etc.)

ANGER

According to the American Psychological Association Society, Anger is an emotion characterized by antagonism toward someone or something you feel has deliberately done you wrong. Anger itself is a normal response. However, the issue is when your anger becomes excessive, uncontrollable, and you lose control of your behavior.

Symptoms:
- Churning feeling in your stomach
- Tightness in your chest
- Changes in behavior
- Feeling nervous
- Increased and rapid heartbeat
- Legs go weak
- Tense muscles
- Feelings of heat
- Have an urge to go to the toilet
- sweating, especially your palms

Strategy
- Think before you speak. It's easy to say something you'll later regret.
- Once calm, express your concerns
- Get some exercise
- Take a timeout
- Identify possible solutions
- Stick with 'I' statements
- Don't hold a grudge
- Use humor to release tension

Herbs that help calm the body and nervous system, and relax the body. Help eliminate toxin buildup and regulate hormones.

Herb Actions:
Adaptogens, Antidepressants, Anti-inflammatory, Detoxification (liver)

Herbs	Methods of Administration
Ashwaghanda (Withania somnifera)	Herb Oils
Chamomile (Matricaria chamomilla)	Teas
Hops (Humulus lupulus)	Tinctures
Lemon balm (Melissa officinalis)	Decoctions
Skullcap (Scutellaria)	Ointments

ANXIETY

Anxiety is a feeling of fear, dread, and uneasiness. Anxiety can be normal in stressful situations such as public speaking or taking a test. Issues arise when anxiety becomes excessive, all-consuming, and interferes with your daily living.

Symptoms

- Sweat
- Feel restless and tense
- Rapid heartbeat
- Having a sense of impending danger
- Panic or doom
- Increased heart rate
- Breathing rapidly (hyperventilation)
- Sweating
- Trembling
- Feeling weak or tired.
- Trouble concentrating

Strategy

- I Peter 5:7 (Prayer)
- Steer clear of alcohol
- Quit smoking
- Keeping active
- Eating well
- Spending time outdoors in nature.
- Spending time with family and friends.
- Reducing stress
- Doing activities you enjoy
- Limit caffeine intake
- Rest
- Eat a balanced diet
- Detox mind and body
- Seek treatment for the root of your anxiety.

Herb Actions:

Herbs that relax strengthen and nourish the nervous system
Sedatives, tension relieving.

Herbs

- Chamomile(Matricaria chamomilla)
- Hops (Humulus lupulus)
- Kava kava (Piper methysticum)
- Valerian (Valeriana officinalis)
- Wild lettuce (Lactuca virosa)

Methods to Administer

- Herb rolled pills
- Teas
- Tinctures
- Decoctions

FEAR

An unpleasant feeling triggered by the perception of danger, real or imagined. Fear is a natural, powerful, and primitive human emotion. Fear is a mechanism that activates our fight or flight response when we are in real danger. This same mechanism helped our ancestors run away from or stand and fight. In our modern world we are dealing with worries and fears regarding how to cope in society. In this case we cannot run away from or physically attack our problems. So we have to be extra careful not to continuously activate our flight or flight response.

Symptoms:
- Sweating
- Trembling
- Dizzy
- Hot flushes or chills
- Shortness of breath or difficulty breathing
- A choking sensation
- Rapid heartbeat (tachycardia)
- Pain or tightness in the chest
- Sensation of butterflies in the stomach

Strategy:
- The only way to deal with fear is to face it
- Pray
- Take time out
- Breathe through panic
- Face your fears
- Imagine the worst
- Look at the evidence
- Talk about it
- Rest
- Exercise

Herbs
- Ashwagandha (Withania somnifera)
- Lavender (Lavandula)
- Lemon Balm (Melissa officinalis)
- Passionflower (Passiflora incarnata)
- St Johns Wort (Hypericum perforatum)
- Valerian (Valeriana officinalis)

Methods of Administration

Teas

Tinctures

Salves

PANIC ATTACKS

A panic attack is a sudden episode of intense fear that triggers severe physical reactions when there is no real danger or cause.

Symptoms:

- Shaking
- Feeling disorientated
- Nausea
- Heart palpitations
- Chest pain
- Rapid, irregular heartbeats
- Dry mouth
- Breathlessness
- Sweating
- Dizziness

Strategy

Immediate:

- Breathe in slowly, deeply and gently through your nose.
- Then breathe out slowly, deeply and gently through your mouth.
- Meditation.

Over-time:

- Stress management
- Healthy diet
- Correct issues of low blood sugar, nutrient deficiency, imbalance in thyroid and adrenals.
- Avoid alcohol
- Reduce caffeine intake
- Physical exercise
- Quitting smoking
- Relaxation techniques

Herbs

Chamomile (Matricaria recutita)
Maca (Lepidium meyenii)
Passion flower (Passifloria incarnata)
Lemon balm (Melissa officinalis)

Methods of Administration

Tinctures
Decoctions

STRESS

Stress can be defined as any type of change that causes physical, emotional or psychological strain. In its natural state stress is a normal psychological and physical reaction to positive or negative situation. This could be a new job or a divorce. The overall goal of our bodys stress response is to It involves a series of physical, psychological, and behavioral reactions that enable people to deal with the stressors and then return to their normal behaviors.

Symptoms
- Irritable, angry, impatient or wound up.
- Over-burdened or overwhelmed.
- Anxious, nervous or afraid.
- Like your thoughts are racing and you can't switch off.
- Unable to enjoy yourself.
- Depressed.
- Uninterested in life.
- Like you've lost your sense of humour.

Strategy
- Fortify the adrenals, brain and metabolism
- Take deep breaths, pray, stretch,and meditate
- Try to eat healthy, well-balanced meals
- Exercise regularly
- Balance hormones
- Protect system against toxins
- Get plenty of sleep
- Avoid excessive alcohol, tobacco, and substance use.
- Remove stress

Herb Actions:
Adaptogenic, Tonic, Nervines

Herbs	Methods of Administration
• Ashwagandha (Withania comnifera)	• Decoctions
• Holy Basil (Ocimum sanctum)	• Teas
• Oats (Avena Sativa)	• Tinctures
• Schisandra (schisandra chinensis)	

UNFORGIVENESS

Unforgiveness is a state of emotional and mental distress that results from a delayed response in forgiving someone. Unforgiveness sets up a domino effect that negatively impacts every part of us, including our emotions, thoughts, spirit, behaviors, and body. Unforgiveness is linked to many health issues such as stress, heart disease, high blood pressure, reduced immune response, anxiety, depression, autoimmune disorders and other health issues.

Symptoms

- Indignation
- Bitterness
- Feelings of stress
- Anxiety
- Depression
- Insecure
- Hardened heart.
- Feels anger
- Resentment
- Impulsive
- Bursts of anger
- Sick

Strategy

- Understand that forgiveness is a process, but must occur for healing to occur.
- Understand that if you refuse to forgive than you hurt yourself more than the person you refuse to forgive.
- Broaden your perspective in life and do something positive for mankind.
- Learn to stay more in the present and not harp on the things in the past.
- Pray
- Rest
- Learn something new

WORRY

Worry refers to the thoughts, images, emotions, and actions of a negative nature in a repetitive, uncontrollable manner. It is feeling uneasy or being overly concerned about a situation or problem. Healthy worry is when a person uses worrying to push them to find a solution or to work hard to achieve their goals.

Symptoms
- Nervous, restless or tense.
- Sense of impending danger, panic or doom.
- Increased heart rate
- Rapid breathing (hyperventilation)
- Sweating
- Trembling
- Feeling weak or tired
- Concentration issues

Strategy
- 1 Peter 5:7
- Eat well-balanced meals
- Limit alcohol and caffeine (can aggravate anxiety and trigger panic attacks)
- Get enough rest
- Exercise daily
- Take deep breaths
- Mindfulness and meditation.
- Deep breathing.
- Practice self-compassion.
- Check in with yourself daily (say out loud what you are feeling)
- Share your fears with trusted friends and family
- Practice gratitude
- Start a journal

Herbs
- Chamomile(Matricaria chamomilla)
- Hops (Humulus lupulus)
- Kava kava (Piper methysticum)
- Valerian (Valeriana officinalis)
- Wild lettuce (Lactuca virosa)

Methods of Administration
- Decoctions
- Teas
- Tinctures

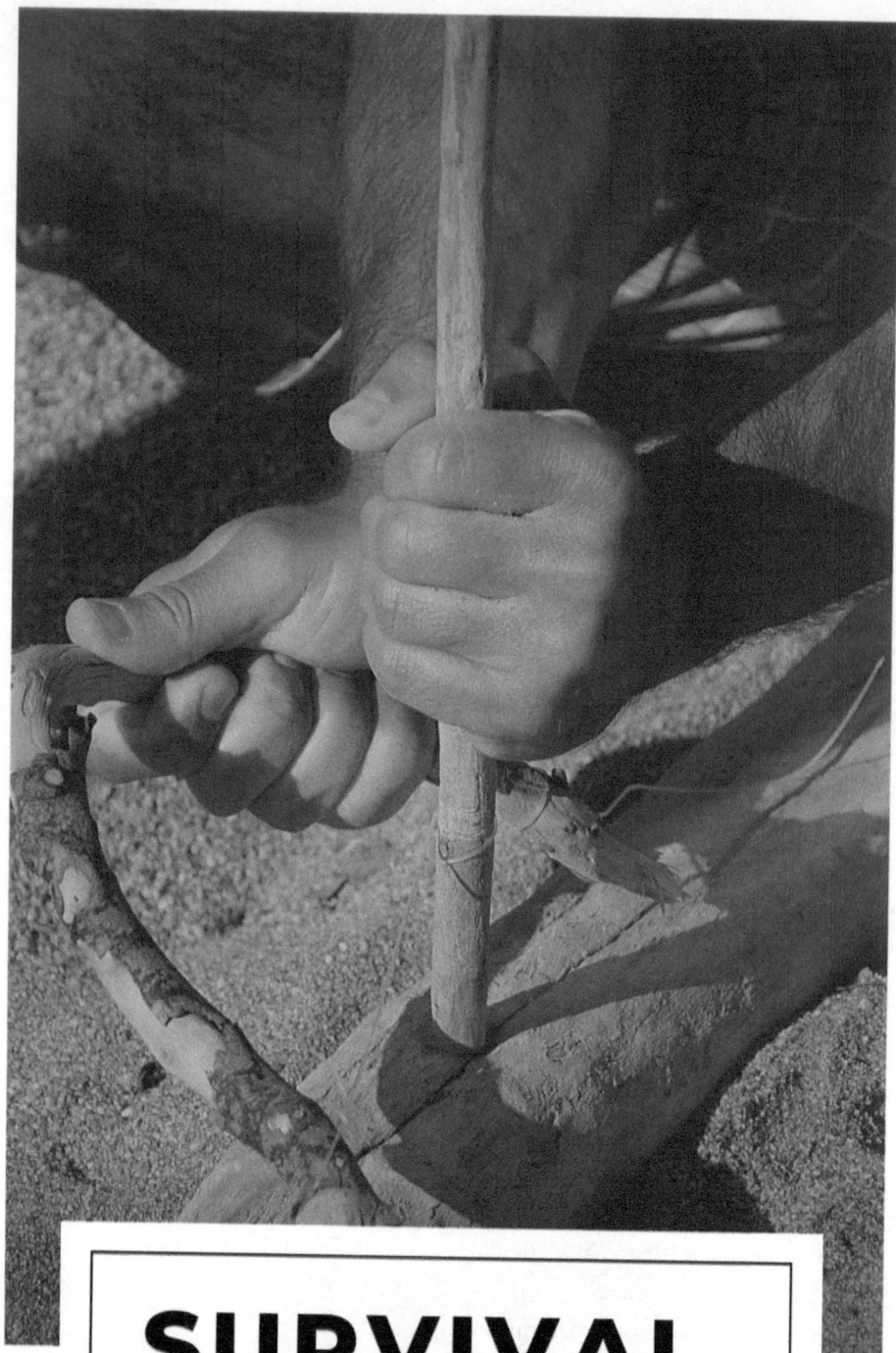

SURVIVAL
SKILLS

SURVIVAL SKILLS YOU SHOULD KNOW

Survival skills are techniques used to help you sustain life in any type of environment whether it be in the wild, suburban or urban areas. These techniques are designed to provide the basic necessities for human life, including water, food, and shelter.

There are many survival skills that you will need to know. I have listed them below:

- Build a fire
- Build a shelter
- Collect and purify Water
- First aid
- Stretch a dollar
- Stretch a meal
- Handle stress and pressure
- Hunt, prepare, and cook food
- How to read a Map
- Navigation skills
- How to protect yourself (weapon building)
- How to forage for your own food

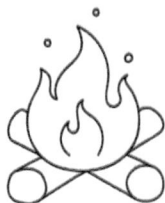

BUILD A FIRE

What is a fire?

Fire is a chemical reaction in which energy in the form of heat is created. The chemical reaction that occurs is called combustion. Combustion happens when fuel or other material reacts quickly with oxygen, giving off light, heat, and a flame.

How is a fire started?:

Fire needs fuel, oxygen and heat, in the right combination in order to occur naturally. Whenever combustible fuel gets in the presence of oxygen at an very high temperature it becomes gas. The flames are an indication that the gas has heated. Oxygen, heat, and fuel are often referred to as the "fire triangle."

How is it used:

A fire can be used for many things such as cooking food, clearing land, generating heat and light, clearing land, and for signaling.

There are many methods to start a fire. However, I am going to talk about two main methods:

Magnifying Glass Method
Bow Drill Method

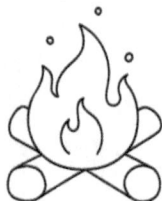

BUILD A FIRE: MAGNIFYING GLASS METHOD

First its important to understand that a fire requires heat, fuel, and oxygen to burn. There are many to start a fire without matches or a lighter. I am going to talk about two ways in this book.

Magnifying Glass (sun glass) Method
Friction Fire (using sticks) Method: Bow Drill

Magnifying glass method

A magnifying glass an great substitute for starting fires in the absence of matches or a lighter.

It makes fire with the help of heat from the sun. You can do this by focusing the glass on the tinder for 50-60 seconds under the sun. The sun rays will pass through the lens of the glass and start producing smoke.

Supplies Needed:
- Tinder (dry paper or wood material)
- Dry sticks and twigs
- A strong and powerful Magnifying glass
- A bright and sunny day

Steps:
- Put the tinder on the ground or appropriate surface. Make sure this surface is directly in the sunlight.
- Hold the magnifying glass over the tinder and hold it in a way that you can see a very small circle of white light on the tinder. Once the tinder starts smoking blow on it until the tinder starts burning.
- Once you establish the fire, put the smallest sticks on the smoldering tinder and then place the larger sticks on the fire until it reaches the size you want.

Final thoughts:

Plants such as Milkweed (Asclepias syriaca L) and the down of Cattail (Typha latifolia) has been found to be extremely flammable.
Birch is also known to be highly flammable.
Tree resin is known to be a fire extender.

FRICTION FIRE: BOW DRILL

Friction fire methods have been used throughout history and continue to be used throughout the world in many cultures. The idea involves grabbing two items and rubbing them together to produce friction, which creates heat.

Supplies Needed:

- 2 inch thick, Fire board/hardwood (wood of medium-hardness, like cottonwood, willow, aspen, tamarack, birch, hickory, cedar, sassafras, sycamore, and poplar)
- Drill
- Spindle (Yucca or same wood as fire board)
- Handhold (piece of hardwood or a rock)
- Paracord
- Tinder

Steps to make a bow drill:

1. **Make the drill:** Cut a straight, dry piece of hardwood 15 inches long. The drill should be as round on one end, sharp point on the other end.
2. **Make handle for the drill:** Use hardwood. The handle should be about 3 in wide by 6 in long by 2 in thick. Carve a hole in the center of the handle about ¼ in deep so that the rounded edge of the drill can fit into it.
3. **Make your fire board:** Choose a piece of softwood (i.e. cottonwood, pine or poplar) that is 6 inches wide by 12 to 18 inches long by 1 inch thick for your fire board. Towards the end of the board cut a v-shaped notch about ½ inch deep into the middle of the board. At the tip of the notch, create a 1/8 inch hole so the drill point to fit into it.
4. **Make your bow:** Create the bow out of a softer wood (cedar, willow, or mulberry) and it should be about 2 feet long and 1 inch thick.
5. **Create your bowstring**: Tie your bowstring (paracord or natural cord of cattail), about 3/8 in wide to the ends of the bow.

* **Remember, use a dead, very dry branch for the spindle and fire board**
* **The bow should be a flexible and as long as your arm.**
* **Fire board should be double the width of your spindle.**

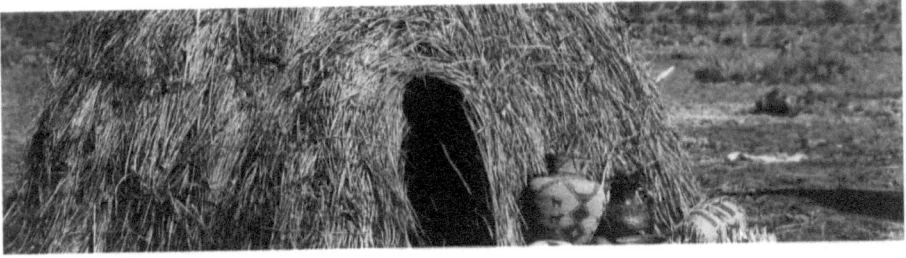

BUILD A SHELTER

Survival shelters can include caves, fallen trees, dugouts, tunnels, debris huts, lean-to's and more advanced structures. Shelters come in many forms and serve a variety of purposes, but one thing is certain, knowing how to quickly build a shelter can save your life.

There are three main forms of natural shelters: the lean-to shelter, the A-frame shelter, and the debris hut.

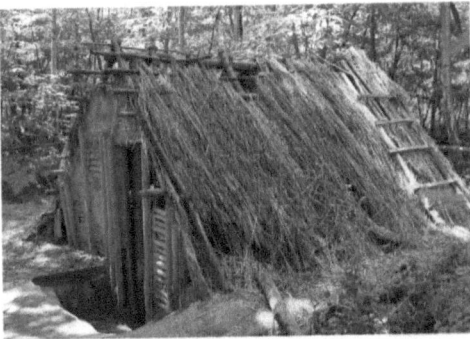

A-Frame

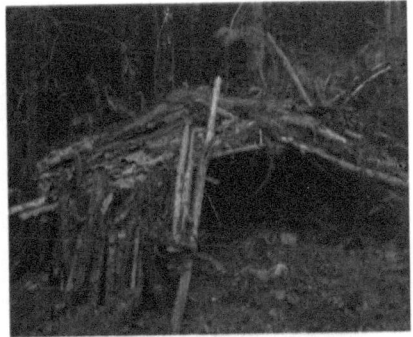

Debris Hut

LEAN-TO-SHELTER

This shelter simply leans on an existing building or against two trees. This shelter is designed to protect you from the wind, snow, rain and debris that might be falling above you.

Time to build: 90 min or less

Supplies:
- Folding Saw
- Cordage (String, rope, paracord, shoelaces, or vine)
- Tarp
- Survival Knife
- Dirt
- Wooden pole (roughly six feet long)
- Poles and sticks (variety of sizes from fallen trees).
- Cuttings (leaves/pine boughs/grass)

Steps:
1. Select a nice flat area with an abundance of natural resources. (Within walking distance to water (lakes or creeks – avoid stagnant water, which attracts bugs))
2. Find two trees that are close together to lean your shelter on (tree's roughly five to seven feet apart over mostly flat ground.)
3. Rest a pole horizontally between your two trees.
4. Secure this horizontal pole with your rope, paracord, string, vine, or shoelaces.
5. Gather more poles of a shorter length to build your wall and rest them against the horizontal pole.
6. Next, use your cordage to secure the poles. Use as many poles and sticks as you can to make sure there are no holes or large gaps.
7. Finally, waterproof your lean shelter by adding more cuttings from bottom to top, layering them upside down so falling water can be channeled away from your shelter.

Keep in Mind:
- Make sure your shelter is facing away from the wind.
- Avoid branches that can catch water or rain and drip inside the shelter.
- Don't build near any hazardous areas.
- Do not leave any branches or supports sticking out, or the shelter can collect water.
- Don't break any live tree branches or kill any plants.

A-FRAME SHELTER

An A-frame is a triangle shaped shelter. It is designed to trap in heat and protect you from the elements on all sides.

Time to build: 1 ½ to 2 hours

Supplies:
- Ridgepole (wood pole to run along the top of your shelter) 2ft longer than your body.
- Side poles (wood)
- Ribs (twigs, branches, etc.)
- Thatching materials (leaves, moss, pine boughs)

Steps:
1. Choose a site. Select a spot with good drainage and steer clear of creek beds.
2. Find a ridgepole and prop it up. The ridgepole is the "backbone" of your shelter. Make sure its sturdy enough to support the weight of your shelter. An alternative can be to prop up your ridgepole between two y-shaped branches or poles. Make sure it is sturdy as you don't want your shelter to fall on you.
3. Next, add side poles for entrance.
4. Add ribs (main branches that will support the walls of your A-frame). Make sure these strong enough to support the weight of your walls. Space them out at least 6 to 12 inches apart along both walls of your shelter.
5. Fill in the ribs. Collect as many sticks, twigs, bushes, and branches as you can find and pile them on and between your ribs.
6. Finally, thatching. Thatching is to make your shelter resistant to the elements (rain, snow, wind etc.). You can use leaves, moss, pine boughs, basically anything water resistant.

Keep in mind:
- The entrance to your shelter should be pointed away from the wind.
- Don't break any live tree branches or kill any plants.
- Don't build near any hazardous areas.
- Do not leave any branches or supports sticking out, or the shelter can collect water.

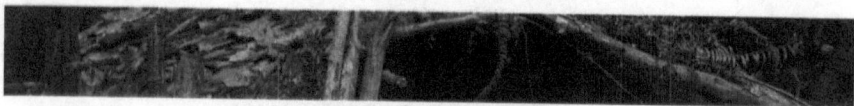

DEBRIS HUT

A debris hut is a simple waterproof hut made of natural materials found in the forest. This three sided structure can be created out of wood, stone, mud, etc.

Time to build: 1-3 hours (depending on the design)

Supplies:
- Sticks
- Debris (moss, leaves, ferns, bark etc.)

Steps:
1. Choose your location carefully. Look for a relatively dry, sunny, and well-drained area with an huge amount of leaves, grass, pine needles, or similar debris.
2. Look for a base to anchor your shelter. This can be a fork in a tree (strongest and easiest option), a stump or a rock.
3. Create your main beam. This beam has to be able to hold up almost 150 pounds of leaves and debris so make sure it's a strong piece of wood.
4. Prop up and secure one end of the beam onto your anchor. Make it high enough for you to get under it.
5. Use your body to measure how wide you want your shelter to be. Keep it tight.
6. Next, gather strong branches to lean them against both sides of the main beam making sure they hit the ground. Create a ribbed effect leaving an opening large enough to be able to crawl into it. Keep the slope steep enough for water to drain off your hut.
7. To keep the debris from falling through the ribbing, weave the finer sticks through your rib frame creating a screen or net look.
8. Lay down your debris at least 2 FEET thick.
9. Next, cover your shelter with some lightweight branches to keep the leaves in place.
10. Pack in insulation. Thickly pack the inside of the shelter with layers of dry materials.
11. Finally, create a way to seal up your entrance.

Keep in Mind:
- Avoid building in animals trails and in areas of running water.
- Build a drainage away from the shelter, so water doesn't begin to pool.
- Build just enough space that you need to keep you warm.
- Keep the ribs tight, so they're better able to hold the leaves.

COLLECT WATER

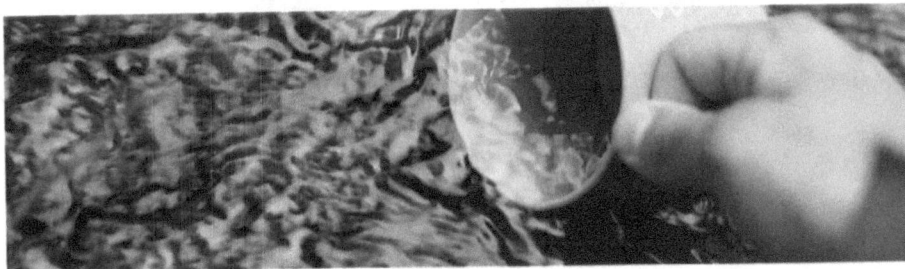

Drinking water is essential to keeping your body functioning properly and feeling healthy. Finding clean and safe water is vital in all survival situations. There are many ways to collect water. When looking for water in the wilderness keep in mind that the higher up the water table you go, the closer you are to the purest water that has not picked up any pollutants dead animals.

No matter were you get your water from, understand that the water may have contaminants that you can't see. The best primary sources of water are those that flow. These are rivers, streams and creeks. If they are not available than you can look to more stagnant bodies of water like ponds and lakes.

Ways to collect water

- Collect rainwater.
- Follow signs of green vegetation or wildlife.
- Melt snow and ice.
- Search for signs of water underground.
- Trap condensation from plants.

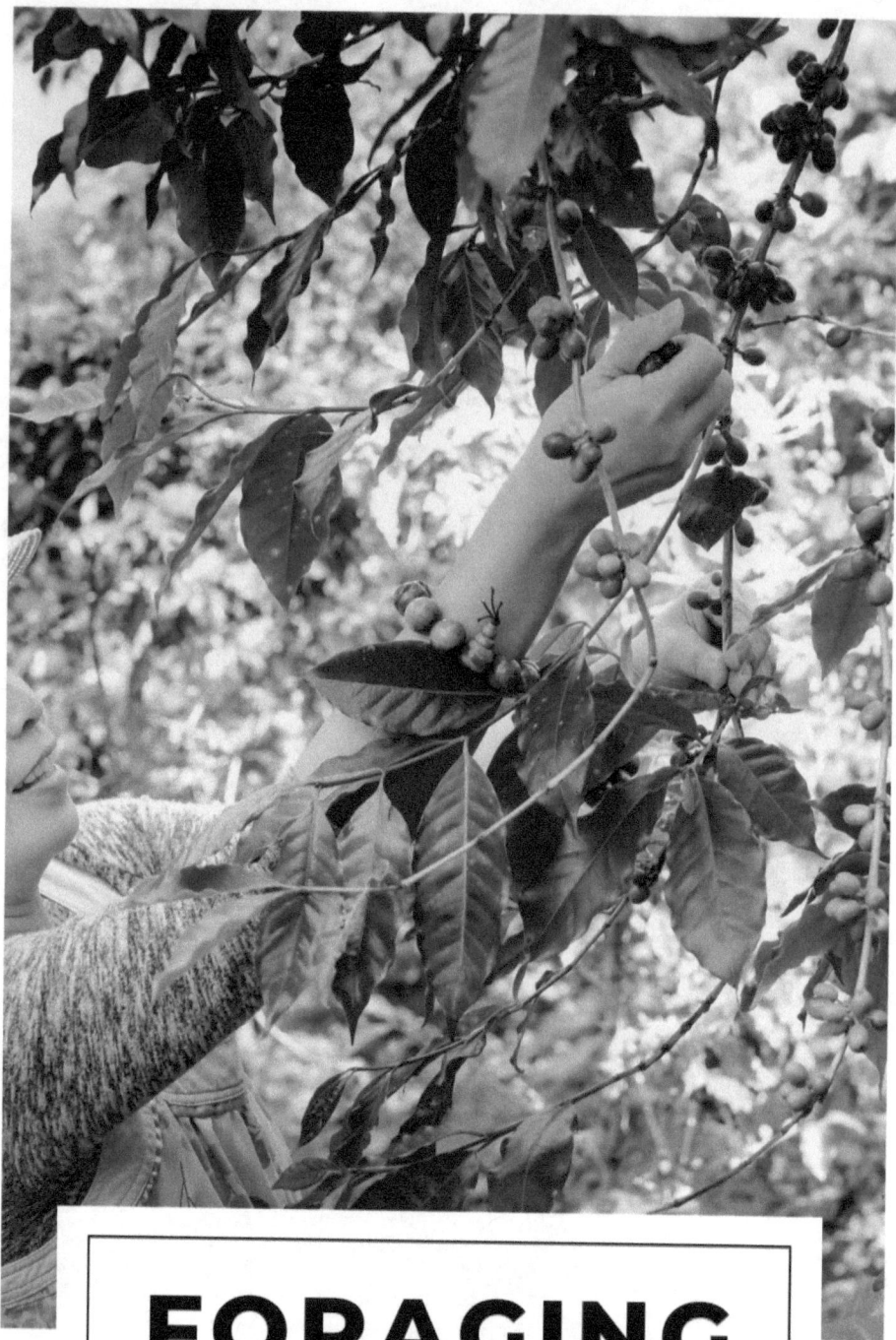

FORAGING

WHAT IS IT?

Foraging is the act of searching, identifying and collecting food resources in the wild. Those include a wide range of plants, mushrooms, herbs and fruits.

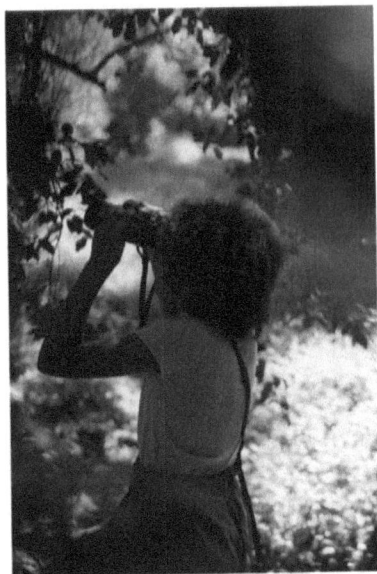

RULES FOR FORAGING

- Know your environment and potential hazards.
- Do not forage around roadways and factories.
- Only forage with permission (If its not your yard.)
- Know the local, state, and federal laws about foraging in your area.
- Take only what you properly identified.
- Be aware of poisonous look a likes.
- Know what plants and insects are invasive and how they spread.

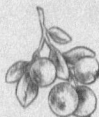

PROPER PLANT ID

What do you need to look at to properly identify plants?

Identifying a plant requires recognizing the plant by one or more characteristics, such as size, form, leaf shape, stem, roots, flower, flower color, odor, and bark, and linking that recognition with a name, either a common or so-called scientific name.

Step 1: Know the scientific and common name of the plant.

Common   Scientific
Wild Yam (Dioscorea villosa)

Scientific Name:

Scientific names are unique plant names used across the world by scientists and other professionals. They are standardized and cannot be changed except by international scientific agreement.

Common Name:

Common names for plants are used by local people. Common names may be totally different from one country to another, from one state to another, and can change as new people move to an area.

Rule of thumb

Start with the scientific name first when looking for plants. This will help minimize confusion especially if you are foraging plants for medicinal purposes.

PROPER PLANT ID

Step 2: Gather field guides to help you find the plants you are looking for.

Get a foraging journal and write down notes on characteristics of the plant you are looking for as well as where to find it.

Step 3: Go find your herbs!

Now that you have the correct names and you have your location picked out, here comes the best part. Finding the plant. You want to look at the following characteristics to help you identify if you have found the correct plant. Always ask yourself, **"does this plant I see have the characteristics that is described in my manual?"**

- **Environment**
- **Stem**
- **Roots**
- **Flowers**
- **Bark**

Environment
It is important to know about the habitat that the plant you are seeking grows in. You would not look for a desert plant in an artic habitat. There are five major habitats, forests, grasslands, deserts, mountains, polar regions and aquatic habitats. Which habitat does your plant grow in?

Stem
There are two basic types of stems. One is green (herbaceous) and another is brown (woody).

Roots
There are two main root systems in plants, fibrous and tap roots. Fibrous (grass) looks like many small fibers hanging off the main root and the tap root (i.e carrot) is one solid root. Observe your plants roots.

Flowers
Pay attention to the shape of the flowers, color, odor and size.

Bark
Pay attention to the bark color, grooves, texture (rough/smooth), peeling direction (horizontal etc.), scales, plates, and fruits or nuts produced.

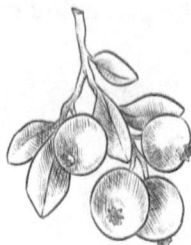

FORAGING TOOLS

There are many foraging tools that can be beneficial however, there are a few key items that you must have on your foraging journey. You don't need an extensive list of supplies. Just the basics. They are:

- Protective clothing
- Cutting tools
- Basket or fabric (linen) bag to carry what you harvested
- Multiple field guides to help you properly identify plants
- Positive and upbeat attitude
- A spirit of gratitude

Some other helpful items include:

- Ruler
- Magnifying glass
- Pine Tree gloves
- Pruning knife and shears
- Compact shovel

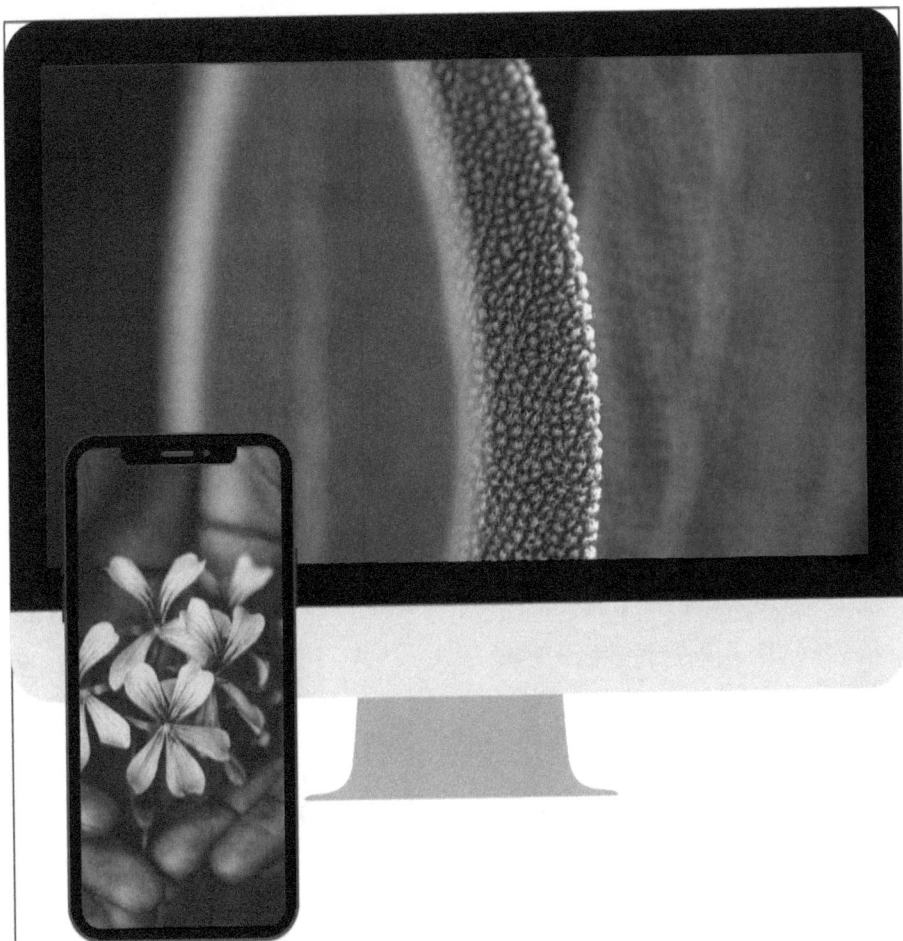

A WORD ON PLANT ID APPS

Just a word of caution, plant ID apps are not always 100% accurate so use caution when using them. They don't take in consideration all aspects of plant id. So be sure to take along your fields guides to help you have additional information that you need to help you correctly identify the plant.

PURIFY WATER

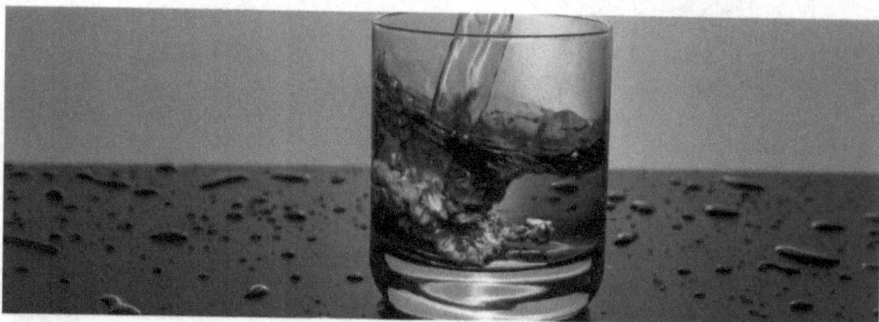

Water purification involves a process that removes germs from water to make it safe for you to drink. Drinking water may contain bacteria, parasites, and viruses which can lead to serious health issues such as diarrhea, cholera and dysentery.

Do not drink water from streams unless you know their source. Springs that are situated on a hillside are usually safe. Areas where cattle graze are not considered safe.

Don't just go off the look of the water. Clear water can contain dangerous bacteria just as muddy water can.

There are several different methods of purifying water.

Boiling:

If there is any doubt, its best to boil your water. Boil it for at least a half an hour.

Iodine:

Mix one drop of Iodine in a quart of water to kill bacteria.

Purification tablets:

Purification tablets normally contain chlorine, chlorine dioxide, or iodine. These chemicals can break down harmful bacteria, viruses, and parasites. Once you put the tablet in the water let it sit for 30 minutes after the tablet has dissolved. It can take up to 4 hours to treat water contaminated with Cryptosporidium. The colder the water is, the less effective the purification tablet will be.

You can eliminate the smell of the water by using small amounts of charcoal boiled in water. This will absorb any odors and make it so that you can taste the water.

STRETCH A DOLLAR

Living paycheck to paycheck? Or just need a change? These days a dollar does not go very far. You can be in a situation where your dollar does not take you as far as you need it to go. So what do you do? Here are a few suggestions:

- Live below your means
- Cut the fat
- Prioritize priorities
- Budget
- Coupon
- Drink water
- Food bank
- Purchase stuff on sale
- Do it Yourself (DIY)
- Dine in

Live below your means
Living below your means is making sure that you have just enough house to live in, a decent car to get you around and you spend money mostly on necessities. You are not living in a home when you can only afford an apartment.

Cut the Fat
Take a look at your expenses and determine where you can make cuts. When money is low you should only be paying necessities (rent, mortgage, car note, food, etc)

Prioritize the priorities
Take a look at your budget. What is the items that you must have in your budget?

Budget
Determine how much money you have coming in and develop a budget around your income.

Coupons
This is not just for old ladies and housewives. Couponing can be for anyone. Those extra savings add up.

Drink water
Drinking water is not only healthier, it can also save you money as well. Juice, sodas, and teas add up.

Food Banks
If you ever get in a situation where the money for food is not available, check your local pantry's and food banks to get some food until you can get back on your feet and once you do.

Purchase stuff on sale
This will help you save a few dollars. Shop for clothes for the next season in the off season.

Do it yourself
If you don't have money to fix things around the house or to have certain things, than learn how to create them for yourself. I've learned a ton from YouTube University.

Dine in
Cooking at home can not only stretch your dollar, it can also be healthier as well. You want that gourmet salmon dinner? Well make it at home for a fraction of the cost.

STRETCH A MEAL

Your check does not come until the 15th and its the 1st of the month. You paid all the pertinent bills and you only had a few dollars left for food. You bought a few staple items but are unsure about how to stretch what you purchased. Sound like you? What do you do?

Purchase foods that stretch

No matter what the situation is you will want to have these staples on hand if ever you need to stretch a meal. These items go far and are bulky, keeping you fuller longer.

Foods that stretch

- Rice
- Beans
- Vegetables
- Oatmeal
- Lentils
- Pasta
- Flour
- Cornmeal

Prepare meals that stretch

Not everyday you will have a meat option, or on some days you might have two chicken thighs to split between a family of six. How can you make this work? You create meals that can stretch. These meals require few ingredients and can stretch.

Meals that stretch

- Casseroles
- Chilis
- Bakes
- Soups
- Rice dishes
- Stir fry
- Vegetables
- Anything with potatoes

Final Tips:

- Meal plan
- Use animal bones to make broths and gravies.
- Buy produce on sale and in season.
- Buy foods whole.
- Buy in bulk when possible.
- Make meat the accent.
- Cut out excessive snacking
- Reuse left overs
- Check clearance section
- Shop multiple stores to find deals.

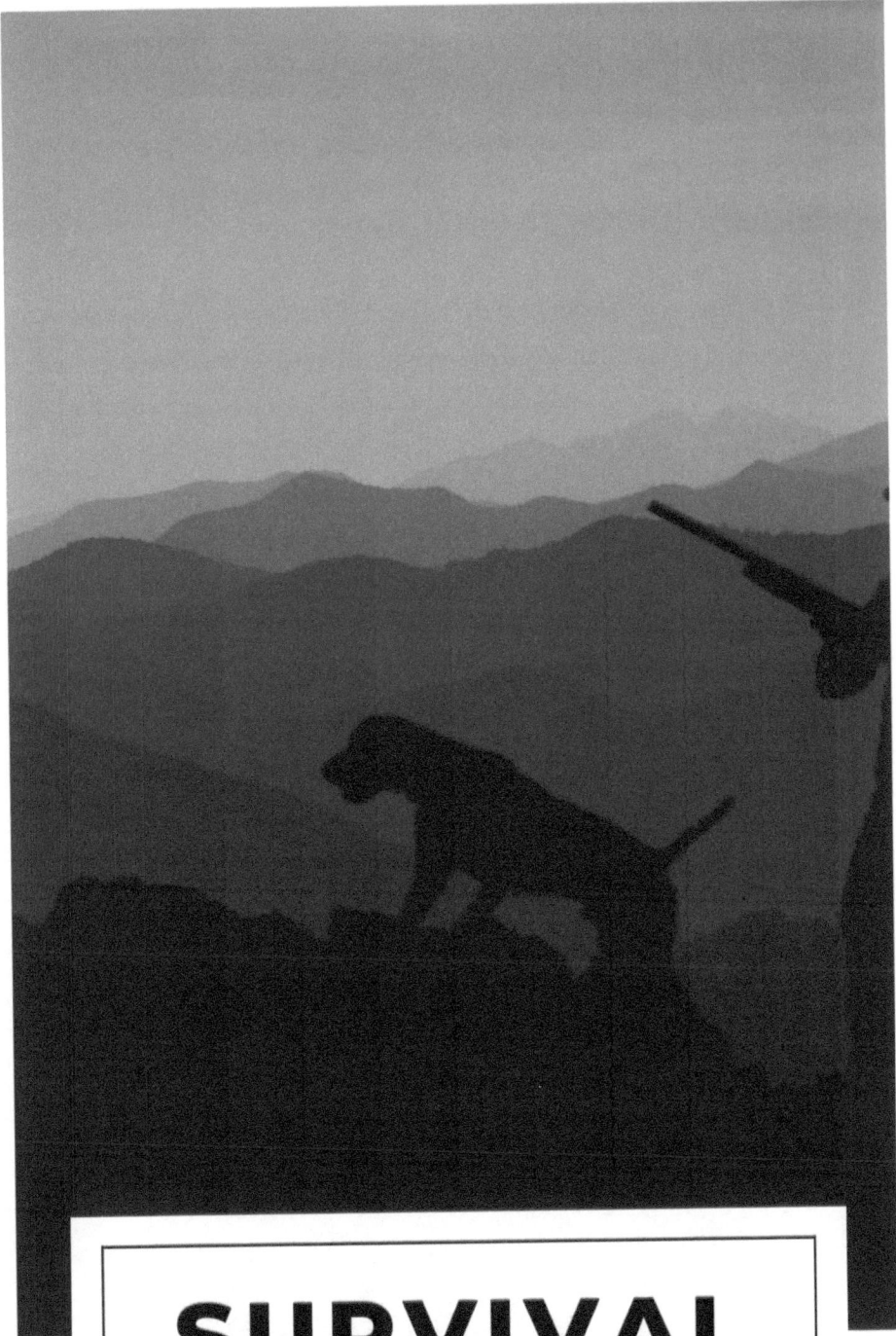

SURVIVAL
HUNT, PREPARE, AND COOK FOOD

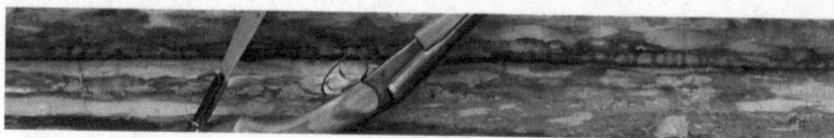

HUNTING 101

To endure the extreme conditions of a survival situation, animal fats and proteins should be eaten regularly, and survival hunting is an essential skill. These situations tend to drain a person's energy. Inclement weather forces your body to metabolize calories at a faster rate so you can stay warm, and perform the physical tasks needed. Most people who get stuck in the wilderness would mess around and starve to death. You don't have to be one of them. Know what grows and is walking around you that is edible so that you don't be one of those people.

Consuming calories from wild edible animals that you got from hunting are an effective way to keep your internal fire going. Every pond, stream, lake, creek, and countryside has animals and wild life that you can eat if the need arose.

In the wilderness, the most practical and wildly accessible wild animals are small game, fish, reptiles and amphibians, and invertebrates. These animals make up for their size with the high numbers of them that you can find. These animals also require very little weapon technology to hunt. you can catch some with your bare hands.

Lakes and streams provide fish, frogs, and crayfish. The woods and fields provide many smaller animals such as woodchucks, rabbits, raccoons, squirrels, and game birds.

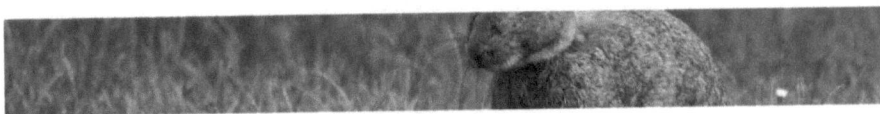

SMALL GAME

Types
- Rabbits and hares, including cottontail, jackrabbit, and snowshoe hare.
- Squirrels, including gray, red, and fox squirrels.
- Prairie Dogs, porcupine, bevers, and raccoons.
- Marmots, groundhogs, woodchucks.
- Muskrats and beavers.

How to hunt

Tool Options
- Slingshot
- Bow and Arrow
- Traps/Snares

Traps
Tie a small loop and pass the end of some wire or string through it to make a loop noose. Put the snare in front of the animal den. If using string, you'll have to use some sticks to prop the noose open. When the animal exits the den, its head will get stuck in the noose.

How to prepare
A simple way to skin small game is to cut the skin around their middle and pull off one side of skin towards the tail and the other towards the head. Then chop off the head and feet.

How to cook
WASH YOUR MEAT! You can either fry or broil the game whole. If the meat is dry, baste with a fat. Older rabbits should be marinated for a day then cooked. Used herbs and spices to flavor the meat.

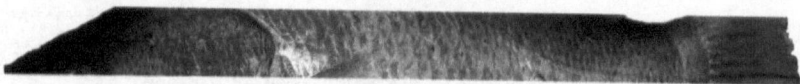

FISH

Types

- Black Bass (Largemouth, Smallmouth)
- Bluefish
- Salmon
- Trout
- Crappie
- White Bass, Striped Bass, and Striped-Bass Hybrids.

Tools

- Hook, line and sinker
- Fishing rods
- Fishing reels
- Fishing bait
- Bite indicators
- Spears
- Nets
- Traps

Traps

Moving Fish Trap- A casting net, also called a throw net, is a net used for fishing.
Funnel Basket Fish Trap (Fastest Method)- A basket used to trap fish with a funnel-like entrance

How to prepare

Step 1: Clean, remove scales, skin guts (do not eat these), and bones.
Step 2: Fillet the fish or create fish steaks

How to cook

Place on grill, camp fire, or bake (if applicable). It takes about 10-15 minutes to cook fish thoroughly. The fish is cooked completely when it easily flakes apart with a fork and is no longer translucent.
**Watch out for sharp teeth, fins, spikes, and barbs hat can cause severe punctures.

SURVIVE

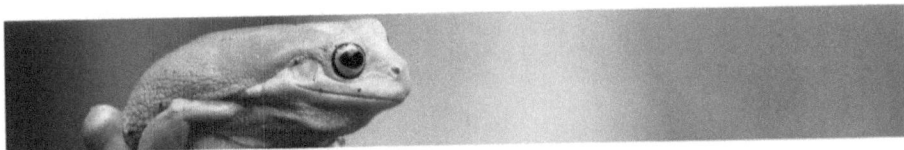

AMPHIBIANS

Amphibians are cold-blooded animals - frogs, toads, salamanders and newts .

Types
- Bullfrogs
- Leopard frogs
- Toads
- Salamanders

Tools
Use a net with a handle and an 18 in (46 cm) hoop to catch frogs. Make sure the webbing of the net is small enough so that a frog cannot escape from it.
Wire fish baskets
Bow and arrow

How to prepare
- First, cut off the feet.
- Slicing the skin around the waist.
- Just take the pliers and grab the loose skin on the back. Anchor the animal with one hand and pull off the skin with the other.
- Use the shears to chop the legs off right at the waist.
- Cut to separate the legs and trim any organ looking bits around the legs.

How to cook
Season your amphibians, wrap them in foil or place them on a stick and heat up over fire. Grill for about 4 minutes. Turn over the legs and brush the other side with the baste mixture. Grill for another 4 minutes or until the internal temperature is at 160°F .

Caution: Some salamanders are toxic. Newts in the genus Taricha can be deadly poisonous, so use caution.

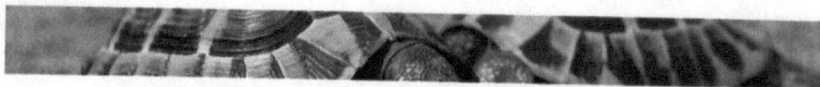

REPTILES

Any of a group of cold-blooded air-breathing vertebrates (as snakes, lizards, turtles, and alligators) that usually lay eggs and have skin covered with scales or bony plate.

Types
- Turtles
- Snakes
- Crocodiles
- Alligators
- Lizzards

Tools
Turtles- Turtles must be killed with a bow and arrow, firearm, or trap.

Snakes- Trap it by its head with a Y-shaped stick and then decapitate it with a knife.

Crocodiles- Can be shot in the head, and if they are below 2m in length, they can be bludgeoned to death with a hammer or other tool.

Alligators- Harpoons and crossbows are popular weapons used to attach a restraining line to an alligator.

Lizards- Use a large box with an open top, some plastic wrap, and food/bait to attract the lizard.

How to prepare
- Remove the skin and clean the reptile
- Cut down the tail, the bone being a guide to open up the tail.
- Remove the white fat inside the tail (alligator).
- Remove the fat
- Hang the turtle by the tail to bleed it. Boil the turtle to remove it from its shell.

How to cook
Cook over fire or pan sear. Cook until internal temperature in the tail reaches 165 degrees on an instant read thermometer about 4 1/2 hours total. Turtles can be cooked for 10-15 min over fire. Cook all meat until tender.

EDIBLE PLANTS: SHOOTS AND LEAVES

Nature has provided us the food we need to survive. We only need to be able to identify it. Many trees have leaves that are delicious in the spring when they first unfold. They can be an interesting and useful addition to spring salads, stir-fry's, and soups.

- **Dandelion (Taraxacum)**- Boil leaves and can be served like spinach or salad.
- **Chicory (Cichorium intybus)**- Young leaves can be consumed raw or boiled as greens.
- **Milkweed Shoots (Asclepias syriaca L.)**- Boil young shoots and young seed pods.
- **Mustard (Brassica nigra)**- Young leaves can add flavor to all greens.
- **Burdock (Arctium)**- Shoots can be eaten raw, stalks can be fried and boiled.
- **Clover (Trifolium)**- Young plants eaten raw.
- **Young grapevine shoots (Vitis vinifera)**- Young shoots cooked in water and grapes can be boiled into jelly.
- **Purslane (Portulaca oleracea)**- Used as an herb or salad.
- **Skunk Cabbage (Symplocarpus foetidus)**- Young shoots boiled and the roots roasted.
- **Common Plantain (Plantago major)**- Shoots can be boiled and eaten as greens.
- **Mesquite (Prosopis)**- Pods have sweet pulp, with hard seeds. Raw beans are pounded into meal.
- **Screw Bean (Prosopis pubescens)**- Can be ground into meal or can make a drink.
- **Passion fruit leaves (Passiflora edulis)**-Passion fruit leaves can also be cooked into soups, curries, stir-fries, pasta, and quiches.
- **Pepper Leaf (Piper)**- Boil the leaves and with salt for the winter months using them in dishes to make braises, soup, and stir fry.

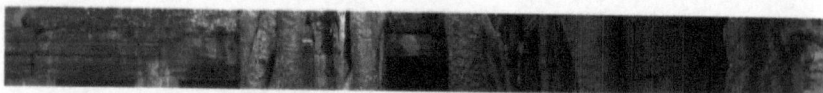

EDIBLE PLANTS: ROOTS

Most plants store their energy in their roots. During the growing season the plant produces as much food and energy as it can, and stores it in the roots. That means wild edible roots are full of energy and nutrition. They tend to be more starchy and filling than the leaves.

- **Arrowhead (Syngonium podophyllum)**- You can cook this root with meat.
- **Cattail (Typha latifolia)**-Can be roasted or boiled.
- **Great Bulrush (Schoenoplectus tabernaemontan)**- Can be eaten raw or cooked. Dry and pound into a sweet flour.
- **Indian Turnip (Arisaema triphyllum)**- Bake, boil, roast or pound into a flour.
- **Ground Nut (Arachis hypogaea)**- Can be boiled or roasted.
- **Indian Cucumber (Medeola virginiana)**- Can be eaten raw. Cucumber in taste.
- **Turk's-cap Lilly (Lilium superbum)**- Bulbs used to thicken stews.
- **Florida Arrowroot (Zamia integrifolia)**- Flour can be made from this root.
- **Biscuit root (Lomatium)**- Celery flavor pounded into flour (watch out for poisonous species).
- **Bitter root (Lewisia rediviva)**- Boiling is the best option.
- **Yellow Adder's Tongue (Erythronium americanum)**-Dry or roast.
- **Chicory Root (Cichorium intybus)**- Is excellent for turning into coffee
- **Camas (Camassia)**- Bulbs can be cooked. They have a chestnut flavor.
- **Chufa (Cyperus esculentus)**- Used to make drinks similar to almond milk.
- **Sand Food (Pholisma sonorae)**- Eaten raw or roasted.
- **Burdock Root (Pholisma sonorae)**- Can be eaten raw or they can be roasted.
- **Sego Lilly (Calochortus nuttalli)**- Sweet corms which can be roasted or steamed.
- **Golden Club (Orontium)**- RIpen seeds can be boiled several times.
- **Man-of-the-earth (Lpomoea pandurata)**- Cousin to the sweet potato, needs to roast for a long time.
- **Toothwort Crinkleroot (Cardamine diphylla)**- Spicy flavor can be eaten like radishes.
- **Jerusalem Artichoke (Helianthus tuberosu)**- You can eat them raw or cooked. They can be mashed, roasted, sautéed or dried and ground into flour.
- **Kudzu (Pueraria montana)**- Can be eaten lioke other root vegetables. Roots can be dried and ground into a powder, to use as breading for fried foods or to thicken soups and sauces.

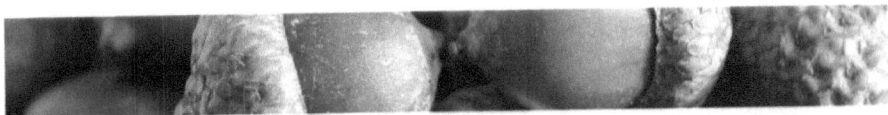

EDIBLE PLANTS: NUTS AND SEEDS

Wild nuts are abundant and nutrient-dense food in the wild packed with natures protein source. Late summer and early fall are the best times to harvest nuts.

Edible Acorns
Sweet enough to eat raw, but is best roasted or boiled and dried. Can be either eaten as a nut, or ground into meal or flour.

White Oaks: Live Oak, Sand Live Oak, White Oak, Swamp Chestnut Oak, Post Oak, Overcup Oak, Chinkapin Oak, Bluff Oak, Bluejack Oak, Blackjack Oak.

Red Oaks: Shumard Oak, Laurel Oak, Turkey Oak, Southern Red Oak, Water Oak, Myrtle Oak, Black Oak.

Water Chinquapin (Nelumbo lutea)- The tubers and the vertical shoots/stems are edible. Can be eaten like peas.

Hickory Nuts(Carya)- Nuts are crushed and placed in boiling water with shells. Oily milk that rises to the top is used for cream or butter.

Beechnut- Oil is shelf stable and has a sweet taste that last for ten years.
Pinon Nuts- Pine seeds that can be roasted.

Chia (Salvia columbariae)- Ground into meal with hot or cold water.

Hog Peanut- Edible peas.

Wild Rice- Cooked as a rice and added to soups.

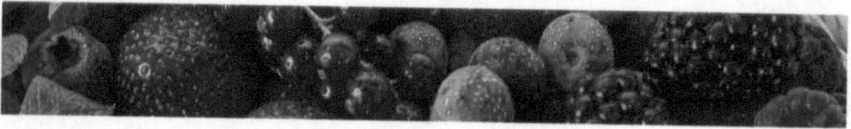

EDIBLE PLANTS: FRUITS

Edible wild berries and fruit are some of the most rewarding things to find when you're out foraging wild edible plants. Unlike roots and greens, wild berries and fruits often don't require preparation and cooking. That makes them very accessible for beginners and provide a sweet bit of instant gratification. Wild fruits within the same genus tend to prefer similar habitats, which means when you stumble onto a patch of wild berries there are likely other similar tasty edibles nearby.

How can you tell if a wild fruit is edible? Look at the:

- Color: Is it dark, blue, red?
- Pulp Texture: The feel of the pulp.
- Pulp Color: The interior color may match the skin color or be different.
- Seed Number: Some species have only one seed while others have many.
- Seed Color: The seed color should be right for that species.
- Seed Size: Are there big seeds, little seeds, or seeds in the middle?
- Seed Shape: Are the seeds round, pointed, oblong, curved, flat.

Berries found in the wild

- Apples and Crabapples (Malus sp.)
- Aronia Berries or Chokeberries (Aronia sp.)
- Autumn Olive (Elaeagnus umbellata)
- Barberry (Berberis sp.)
- Bearberry (Arctostaphylos uva-ursi)
- Blackberry (Rubus sp.)
- Blackcaps or Black Raspberries (Rubus oc.)
- Black Cherry (Prunus serotina)
- Spanish Bayonet (Yucca aloifolia)
- Strawberry (Fragaria virginiana)
- Service Berry (Amelanchier ar.)
- Choke Cherry (Prunus virginia.)
- Mountain Ash (Sorbus ameri.)
- Rose Hips (Rosa canina L)
- Salal (Gaultheria shallon)
- Hawthorn (Crataegus)
- Manzanita (Arctostaphylos)
- Elderberry (Sambucus)

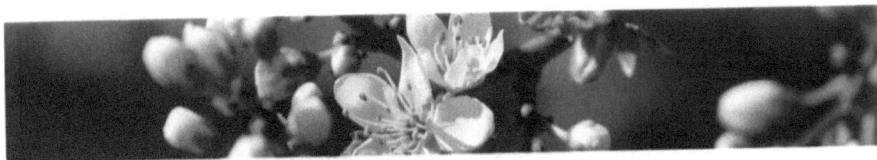

EDIBLE PLANTS: BUDS

The bud is the young part of a plant that's almost ready to flower or unfold new leaves. It is a small pointed bump that appears on a tree or plant and develops into a leaf or flower.

Edible Buds

Basswood Buds (Tilia americana)- Buds can be eaten raw or cooked.

Red Bud Flowers (Cercis canadensis)- Buds and their pods are pickled or fried.

Palmetto (Sabal Palmetto)- Can be cooked or eaten raw.

Joshua Tree Buds (Yucca brevifolia Engelm)- These buds have a high sugar content and can be roasted on coals.

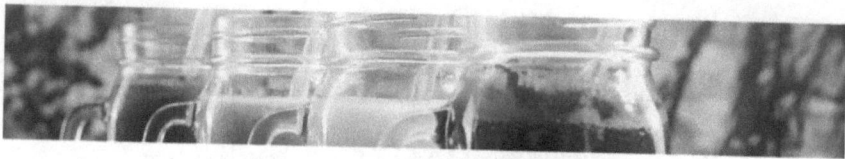

EDIBLE PLANTS: DRINKS

Tired of drinking water? Want to mix things up? Nature also has the answer. You can use plants to make teas and ciders.

Herbal Teas:

Sumac (Rhus)- Boil the fruit of the dwarf and staghorn sumacs to create a lemonade.

Manzanita (Arctostaphylos) - Cider can be made using the berries.

Sassafras (Sassafras albidum)- Cut the root to make a tea.

New Jersey (Ceanothus americanus)- The leaves of this shrub can be boiled to make tea.

Spice-Bush (Lindera benzoin) - The twigs can be boiled into a tea.

Wintergreen (Gaultheria procumbens)- Leaves can be boiled in water to make a tea.

Cherry or Black Birch (Betula lenta L)- Tea can be made by steeping the twigs and bark.

Yarrow (Achillea millefolium)- The leaves can be boiled into a tea.

Chicory (Cichorium intybus)- Roots are boiled in water to make a tea.

Herbal Coffees:

Sunflower (Helianthus)-Roasted sunflower seeds grounded into coffee.

Kentucky Coffee Tree (Gymnocladus dioicus)- Seeds roasted and ground into coffee.

Purple Avens (Geum rivale)- The root stalk and leaves made into a decoction.

Corn (Zea mays)- Coffee from roasted corn.

Dandelion (Taraxacum)- Made from roasted dandelion root parts.

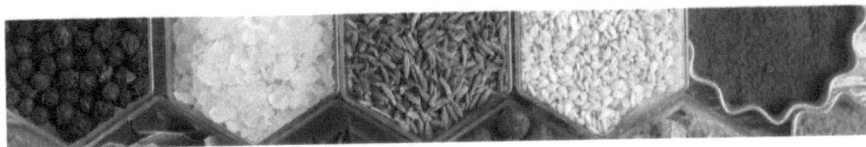

EDIBLE PLANTS: SEASONINGS AND FLAVORINGS

Our ancestors used natures seasonings to add flavor to the dishes they created. There are many plants that can be used to add additional flavor to our meals.

Seasonings

- Colt's foot Salt (Tussilago farfara)- Burn leaves to create salt.
- Spice bush (Benzoin aestivale)- Seasoning made from dried berries.
- Chili Pepper (Capsicum annuum)-Peppers were dried and ground.

Flavorings

- Mint (Mentha spicata)- Used in drinks, stewed meats, and boiled to clean meat.
- Spearmint (Mentha spicata)- Mixed in vinegar and placed on meat.
- Peppermint (Mentha piperita)- Used in candy making and flavoring.
- Wild Ginger (Asarum canadence)- Used the roots as flavorings.
- Wintergreen (Gaultheria procumbens)- Flavoring
- Sweet Bay (Persea borbonia)- Used to flavor soups.
- Cherry Birch (Betula lenta)- Sweet flavoring. Twigs and and buds used to flavor food and drinks.
- Sassafras (Sassafras albidum)- Leaves dried and powdered to use as thickeners and flavorings.
- Spice Bush (Lindera benzoin)- Berries and leaves are dried and powered to flavor meats, stews, and soups.
- Wild Leek (Allium tricoccum)- Bulbs add flavor and can be paired with meats and other vegetables.
- Vinegar- Made from plant juices and saps of maple and birches allowed to ferment.
- Wild Mustard (Sinapis arvensis)- Seeds sprinkled on food to add flavor.

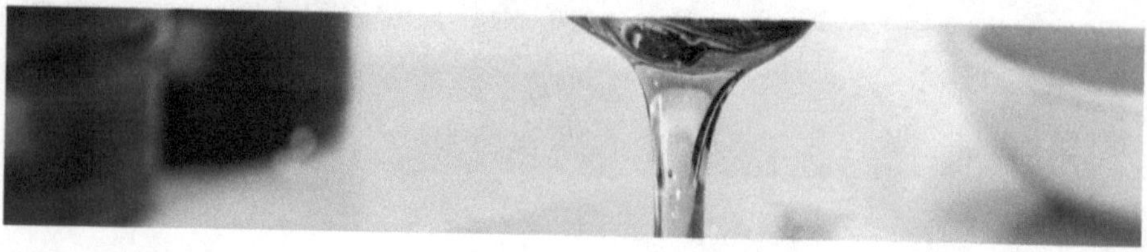

EDIBLE PLANTS: SYURPS AND SUGARS

Did you know that nature provides a way for us to enjoy sweets? Our ancient ancestors knew which plants provided this sweet goodness. Here is a list of natures sugars and syrups.

Maples

Maples are created by boiling sap over a slow fire.

Sugar Maple (Acer saccharum)

Red Maple (Acer rubrum)

Striped maple (Acer pensylvanicum)

Hickory (Carya)

Ash leaf maple (Acer negundo)

Sugar Trees

Sugar Pine (Pinus lambertiana)- Sap that forms lumps.

Milkweed syrup/sugar (Asclepias)- Boiling blossoms extract a sweet syrup.

Butterfly weed (Asclepias tuberosa)- Boiled orange flowers into sugar and syrup.

Bulrush (Scirpus)- Boiling the bruised root to get a syrup.

Mesquite (Prosopis)- Dried and ground into a meal to sweeten meals or cereals.

Screw Bean (Prosopis pubescens)- Boil the pods to get a syrup.

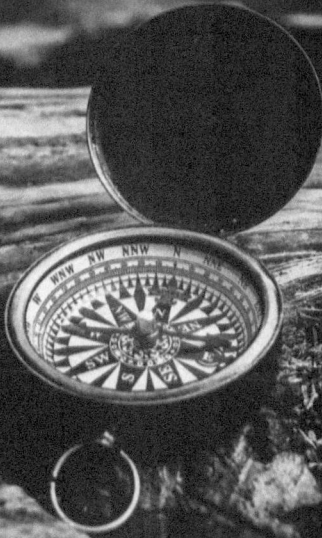

NAVIGATION

MAP READING

Map reading is important survival skill to have. It helps you understand your geographic location portrayed on a map. Always have a good map of the country that you are in or planning to go through. Knowing the features is important when honing your skills of how to read a map. Listed below are important features of a map and an explanation about them.

Types of maps

Topographic Maps- It shows detailed information about the terrain, roads, points of interest and distances.

Road Map-Road maps are a great accessory to bring on a road trip

Tourist Map- They generally show the attractions and points of interest around a city.

Colors on a topographical map

Green- Means areas of vegetation.

Brown- Contour lines showing elevation.

Blue- Water sources (i.e rivers, lakes).

Black- Man made objects, i.e. building or railway.

Red: Major roadways (i.e. highways).

What is on a map?

- Legend
  - Gives a description and guide of the different features and markings on the map.
- Title
  - Tells you what area the map is of.
- Grid References
  - A location on a map, which is found using the north and east numbered line. Grid references are useful for helping a map user to find specific locations.
- The North Arrow
  - This arrow tells you which way is north – it always points to the top of the map.
- Scale
  - The scale will tell you what scale your map is – whether it's 1:25,000 or 1:50,000.The scale is 1 inch to 1 mile.

HOW TO READ A MAP

Knowing how to read a map is just as essential as having one. If you know how to read a map it is rare that you will get lost. Your map will be able to tell you in detail the terrain around you. So, how do you read a map?

Pay attention to contour lines

Contour lines determine the steepness of the terrain. They connect points that share the same elevation indicating the terrain is steep. Where contour lines are further apart there is a gentle slope.

Contour lines also indicate the shape of the terrain. Roughly concentric circles (circles that share the same center) are probably a peak, and areas between peaks are passes.

Index contour lines: Every fifth contour line is a thicker "index" line. At some point along that line, its exact elevation is listed.

Contour interval: The change in elevation from one contour line to the other is the same within the same map. You can find the contour interval for your map in its legend.

Pay attention to the scale

A map's scale tells you how detailed the map is. A 1:25000 scale, for example, means one inch on the map equals 25,000 inches of real-world terrain. A large scale means that the map is showing greater detail and the small scale means that the map has less detail.

Look at the map legend

It contains map-reading clues and navigational info. Start by understanding what each line, symbol and color means. It also has the magnetic declination (information needed to set up your compass).

Practice....Practice....Practice....

COMPASS

A compass is a device for finding direction. How a compass works is by detecting and responding to the Earth's natural magnetic fields. How is the earths magnetic field created? The Earth's core is made of iron that is part liquid and part solid crystal, which is due to the gravitational pressure. It is understood that when there is movement of the liquid in the outer core, this action produces the Earths magnetic field.

Parts of the Compass

The most important part on the compass is the magnetic needle. The needle swings around the compass as you move, however the red end will always point north and the white (or black) end of the needle will always point south. The other parts include:

- **The Compass Body or Housing**: Houses the movable parts of the compass.
- **Direction-of-travel Arrow**: Tells you which direction to point the compass when you're taking or following an angle.
- **Orienting Arrow:** A fixed arrow painted underneath the movable parts of the compass.
- **Compass Needle:** The movable part of the compass that follows the earth's magnetic pull.

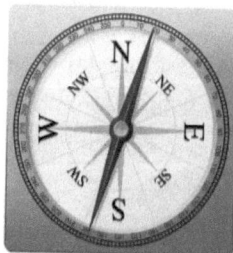

Words of advice: Make sure that when you are using your compass there are no metal, power lines or magnetic objects near it when you read it as they can skew your compass readings. This objects will influence the magnetic needle and give you a false reading.

HOW TO USE A COMPASS

Pick up the compass and hold it flat in front of you. Be sure that the direction of travel arrow points straight ahead. Then, rotate yourself, keeping an eye on the magnetic needle. When the red end lines up exactly with the orienting arrow, stop.

Correcting for Declination

When a compass is used with a map, a correction must be made to allow for declination. Magnetic (compass) north isn't the same as true (Earth) north. The angle between the two is known as declination (magnetic variation). The declination will vary depending on your location and it can gradually change over time as the Earth's tectonic plates shift. You have to adjust your compass to account for the declination otherwise you will be headed in the wrong direction.

How to find the Declination

The quickest way to find the angle of declination is to look at your map. There should be an angle and direction (i.e 10 degrees west). The more updated your map, the more accurate your declination will be.
Once you identify your declination now its time for calculations. For East declination, subtract declination from your compass reading. For West declination, add declination to the true compass reading.

After adjusting your compass for declination, Its time to travel!

Place the corner of your compass's base plate on your current location, then rotate your entire compass until the straightedge forms a line between your location and where you are trying to go.

Next, rotate the bezel until the grid lines on the base plate match the grid lines on the map. Make sure everything lines up.

Read the number that is next to the index line, this is called your bearing.

Holding the compass so that it is level in front of you and rotate your body until the north arrow on the bezel matches the compass's needle.

Your direction-of- travel arrow should be pointing towards your desired destination.

SURVIVE

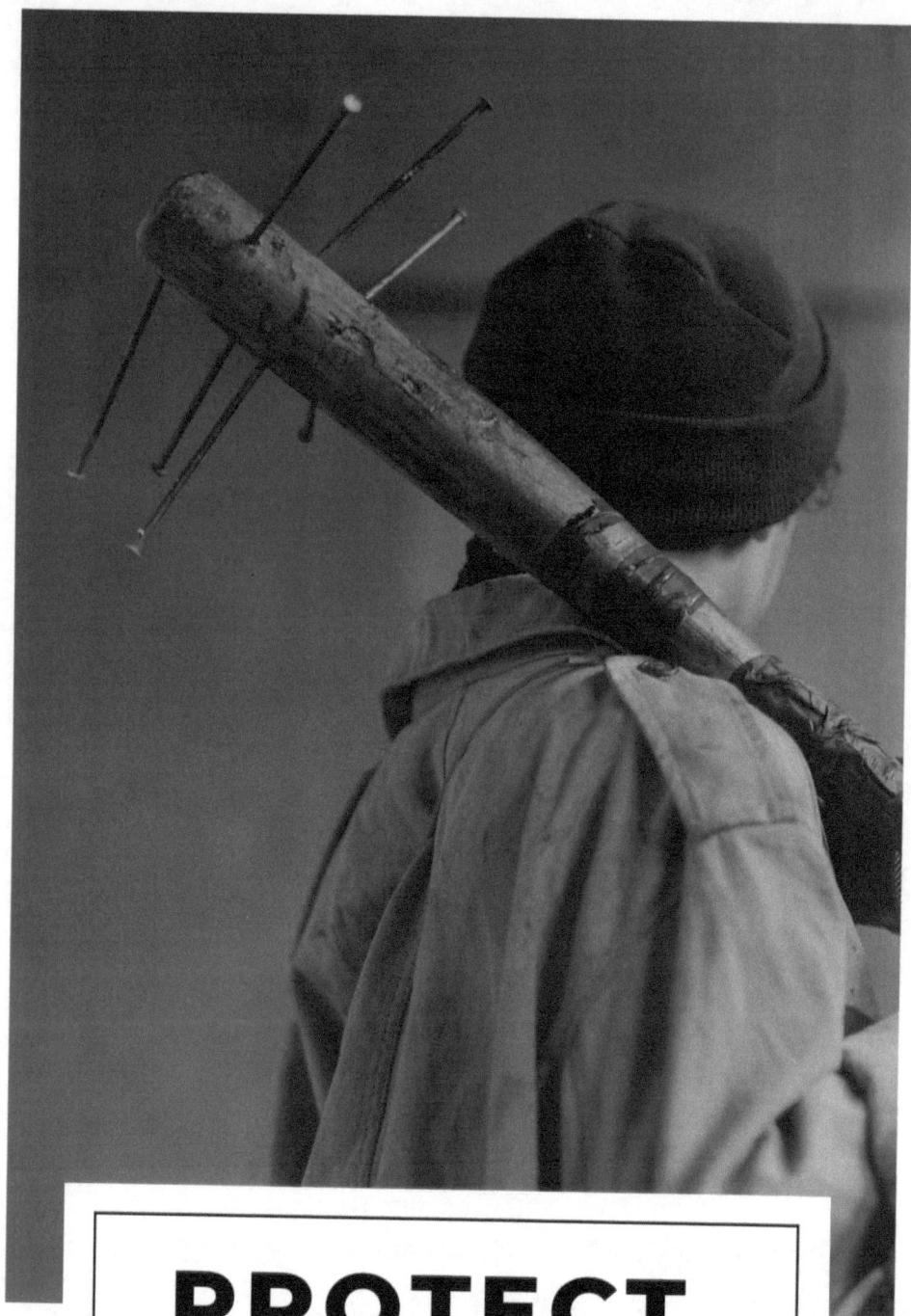

PROTECT
YOURSELF

WEAPON BUILDING

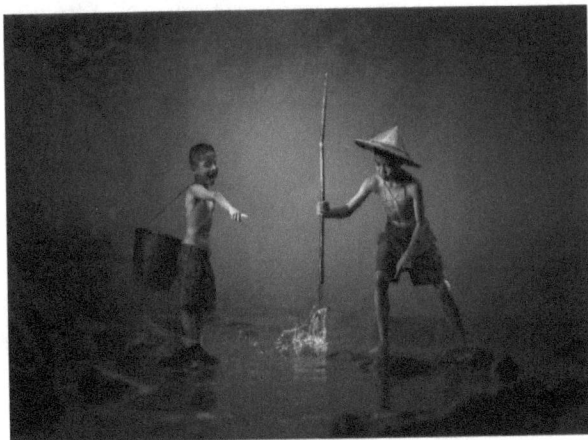

If you are on the earth without an adequate means to defend yourself than you are in trouble. You may say "well i have a gun cabinet stocked full of all the finest weaponry". However, what happens if you no longer have access to your extensive army arsenal? What do you do? I'll tell you.... learn to improvise.

Security is a vital aspect of survival. Weapons give you the ability to not only defend yourself, but to also to kill wildlife for food. In weapon building there are many types of weapons you can make. For the sake of simplicity I am going to outline two main categories of weapons:

- **Blunt-Force Weapons**
- **Piercing Weapons**

Blunt-Force Weapons are simple and can do a lot of damage when used correctly. The club is one of the most well-known weapons in this category. Batons, clubs, Kali sticks, and sling shots also fall into this category. You can easily create these weapons in the wilderness using a solid tree branch. In an urban environment you can use a metal pipe, cast iron skillet, or a wood 2x4.

Piercing Weapons are designed to slash or stab. They include spears,bow and arrows, kubatons, spikes, knives, and swords. If you're in an urban environment, you could use a knife, scissors, letter opener to create spears.

CLUBS

Clubs can not only be used for protection, you can also use clubs to hit animals, such as possums, porcupines, raccoons, and rodents. There are many types of clubs you can create. I will outline a few here.

Types of clubs:
- Simple Club
- Weighted Club
- Sling

Simple Club:
A simple club can be made from a staff or branch. The diameter of it should fit comfortably in the palm of your hand. It should not be too thin or it will break upon impact.

To create:
Grab a knife, cut out a V-shaped notch in the top of your sturdy stick(consider using a straight-grained hardwood if you can find it to create your handle), that has a forked end and put a round rock in between the forked end. Next, use your handmade rope to tie the rock in place.

Weighted Club:
A simple club with a weight on one end. It can be made with a natural weight, such as a knot on wood, or a stone attached to the club.

To create:
Find a stone (one with a slight hour glass shape) that has a shape that will allow you to secure it to the club.
Next, find a piece of wood (a straight-grained hardwood) that is the right length for you. Finally, secure the stone to the handle with cordage. (whatever cord you choose).

There are three techniques for attaching the stone to the handle: split handle, forked branch, and wrapped handle.

Sling Club
Another type of weighted club. A heavy weight hangs 8 to 10 centimeters from the handle by a strong, flexible cord .

To create:
Tie a cord to the wooden pole, leave 2- cm free.
Tie stone or rock to cordage, leave 7.5 to cm from club.

SPEARS

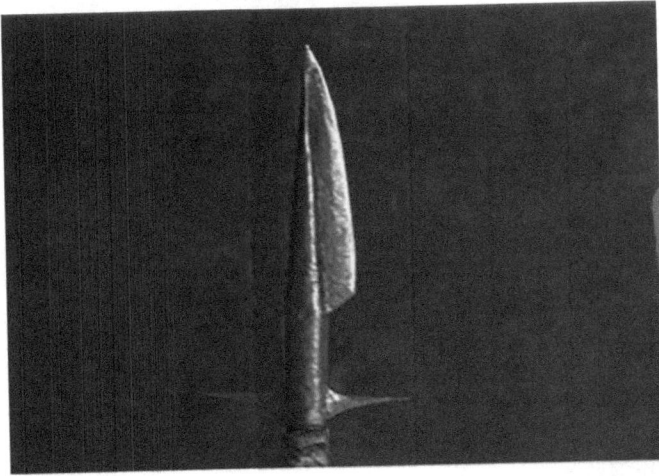

A spear is one of the most versatile weapons. You can use them in a variety of ways such as to catch fish, and attack your attackers while maintaining a safe distance.

Supplies needed:
- A stiff wooden pole approximately one and a half meters in length
- Sharp survival knife (or created survival knife out of rock)
- Shells, bone or metal
- Paracord (or other cordage)

To create:

1. Take your survival knife and create a pointed tip by shaving off the edges near the top.
2. To make the point durable, place the sharp point over a fire while rotating it frequently to harden the tip.
3. If you want to create a spear with a spear blade (made of either metal, wood, bone or shells), attach the spear blade to the shaft using lashing (cordage). You can attach it by splitting the handle, inserting the blade, and then wrap or lash it tightly.

BOW AND ARROW

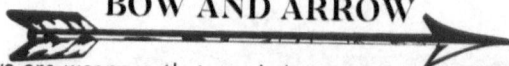

Bow and arrows are weapons that can help you remove attackers by yourself. They're discreet weapons you can use to conduct slient long-range attacks. Arrows also fly at high speeds which makes them effective for eliminating big targets.

Supplies needed:

- A piece of wood (the material must be flexible with the ability to snap back into position quickly. A branch about the size of your pinky)
- 10-foot paracord (can be made from natural materials such as dogbane, milkweed, yucca or nettle)
- Survival knife
- A pocket tool

To create:

1. Carefully chop off the wood and shave off any extra branches using your survival knife.
2. Use the survival knife to shave the side facing towards you. Leave the unshaved side facing towards your target.
3. Be sure to sharpen the tips on both sides so you can tie on the bowstring or paracord.
4. Carve notches at both tips of your bow. The notches should be about one-inch deep.
5. Tie the paracord tightly on both sides then lay your bow on the ground. Make sure both ends rise together at the same time.
6. As for the arrows:

Arrows:
You can use straight shoots from trees such as maple, willow or dogwood. Clear the wood of branches and knots, and taper gradually end-to-end.
The small end of the arrow should be notched for the string and should be large enough for this knock without compromising the strength of the wood on either side. scrape the bark from the wood and then hold over a fire to straighten it out.
The large end of the arrow can be sharpened to a point or notched to accept a point of steel, shell, stone, or bone.

Now take it out and practice...practice...practice...

KUBATON

A kubotan is a five to six inch long stick self defense weapon made of either wood, steel, or any other durable material. This weapon was developed by Sōke Takayuki Kubota in the late 1960s.

How do you use a Kubaton?

You use this weapon for punching and attacking vulnerable parts of an attackers body,. Common areas to target are, the groin, throat, shin, hip, eyes, ankle, or kneecap. This includes any body part that is extremely hard or fleshy as these parts can elicit the most pain in your attacker.

Supplies needed:

- Piece of wood (make sure it can fit comfortably in your hand) about 5-6 inches Long
- Knife
- Cordage for handle

To create:

1. Take the wood and remove branches and ridges.
2. On the wood make marks an inch apart going down the piece of wood.
3. On one end use the knife to create a sharp rounded point.
4. On the other end use the cordage to create a key chain effect.

SLING SHOT

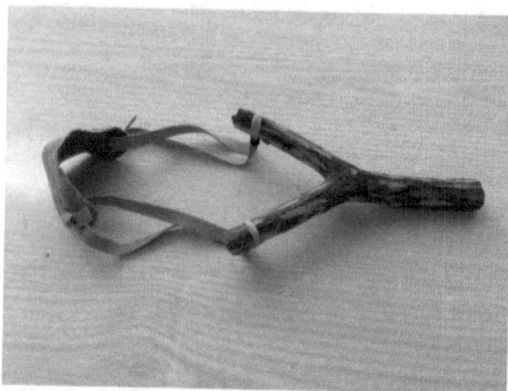

A slingshot is a a forked stick, to which an elastic strap is fastened to the two prongs, and used for shooting rocks, marbles, and metal balls.

A slingshot is a weapon that allows one to hit targets long range, up to 250 feet. It has a variety of ammunition such as rocks, marbles and metal balls. It requires very little training and can be used by children (with supervision) and adults.

Supplies needed:

- A thick fork of branches that has a 2-3 inch diameter
- A piece of leather (3x3)
- Rubber band
- A pair of scissors
- 1 meter of plastic thread

To create:

1. Cut the rubber band into two equal strips (8in long and 3 inches wide)
2. Drill two small holes near the vertical sides of the rectangle.
3. Attach the rubber band strips on both holes of the leather strip. Use bits of plastic thread to firmly tighten the ends so that your rocks don't slip out while you pull the sling shot.
4. Tie the loose ends of the rubber strips to the tips of your fork using your plastic thread.

Test Your slingshot to see if everything is in place.

PEPPER SPRAY

Pepper spray is a spray that contains an inflammatory compound called capsaicin. It causes burning, pain, and tears when it comes into contact with any attacker. This survival weapon can use to disarm one or two attackers at the same time. Its a good idea to add this to your weapon arsenal.

Supplies needed:

- A 100ml spray bottle
- Rubbing alcohol
- Two clean bowls
- 4 tablespoons of spicy powder (ghost peppers, chili powder, or black pepper)
- A plastic/metal kitchen strainer
- Two tablespoons of coconut/olive oil

To create:

1. Put the hot powder into a clean bowl and slowly pour in your rubbing alcohol. Then, cover and let it soak for eight hours for the hot powder to saturate.
2. Next, add the two tablespoons of coconut or olive oil to increase your sprays density.
3. Use your kitchen strainer and carefully sieve the mixture into a clean bowl to trap the solid particles.
4. Pour the homemade spicy solution into a dry 100ml spray bottle and test it on your leg.
5. Finally, store your pepper spray weapon in a cool and dry place to enhance its longevity.

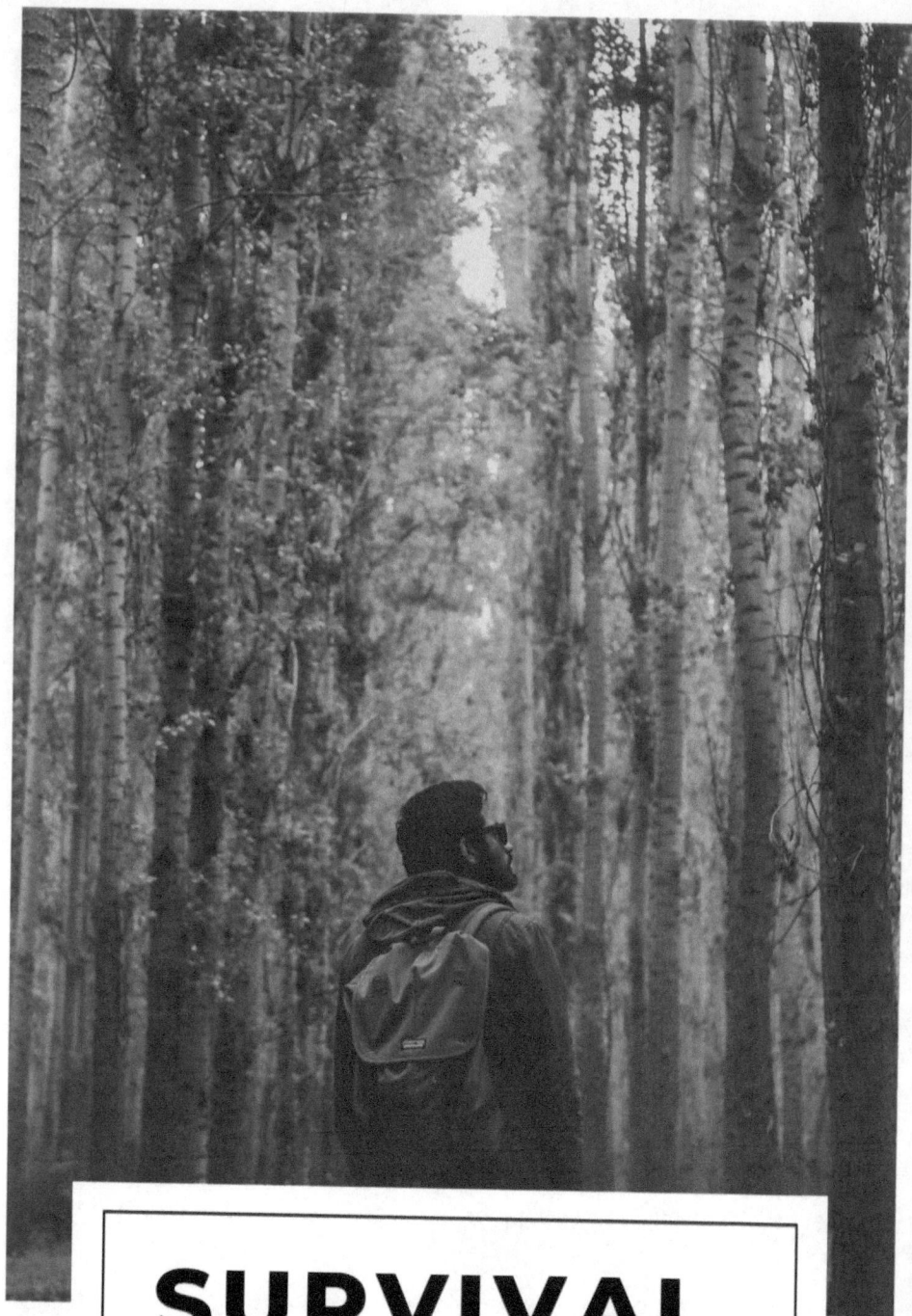

SURVIVAL
KIT

WHAT YOU NEED

Basic First Aid Kit
Antiseptic wipes
Bandage strips
(various sizes and types)
Cold packs
Disposable gloves
Dressings
Duct tape
Elastic wrap
Epinephrine injector
Flashlight and extra
Batteries
Gauze pads (various
sizes).
Headlamp
Personal medicines
Scissors
Tape
Tweezers
Additional First Aid
Supplies
Bandana
Basin for soaks
Butterfly
Bandages
Cloth for
Compress
Elastic bandage
Eye cup
Face mask
Hot water bottle
Hydrogen peroxide
Irrigation syringe
Matches, lighter
Multi-tool
NSAIDs
Povidone iodine
Rubbing alcohol

Scalpel
Self-adhesive bandage
Soap
Steri-strips
To-go bottles
Wildcrafting tools
1½" White Athletic Tape Roll
3" Ace Wrap
2" Ace Wrap
Cravat
Wound Wash
Assorted Band-Aids (Small to
Large)
SAM Splint
Hand/Alcohol Wipes 5 of each
type
Metal, fine point tweezers 1
Ultra-Thick Ziplocks 4 x 4 (for
bandaids, etc.)
Bandage Scissors
Metal Hemostats
Scalpels
18 ga. needle
20cc Syringe (irrigation)
USP grade Charcoal, 4 oz.
(high medical grade for both
external infection poultices
and internal poisoning)
Cold Pack
Nitrile Gloves
Kerlix Bandage Roll
Self-Adhesive, 2" wrap
Olaes Modular Bandage
Casualty Blanket (and shelter)
Mini dark glass bottles
Pipettes
Essential Oils
Herb products

Honey (Preferably
Manuka Grade 12+ or
greater),
4 ounces Bentonite Clay
Q-Tips
Roll of Dental Floss
Hydrogen Peroxide
Aspirin/Motrin
Headlamp,
Small magnifying glass
Fresnel lens
Toenail Clippers
Duct Tape (Small, hand-
made roll)
Abdominal or large
bandage
Personal Gear

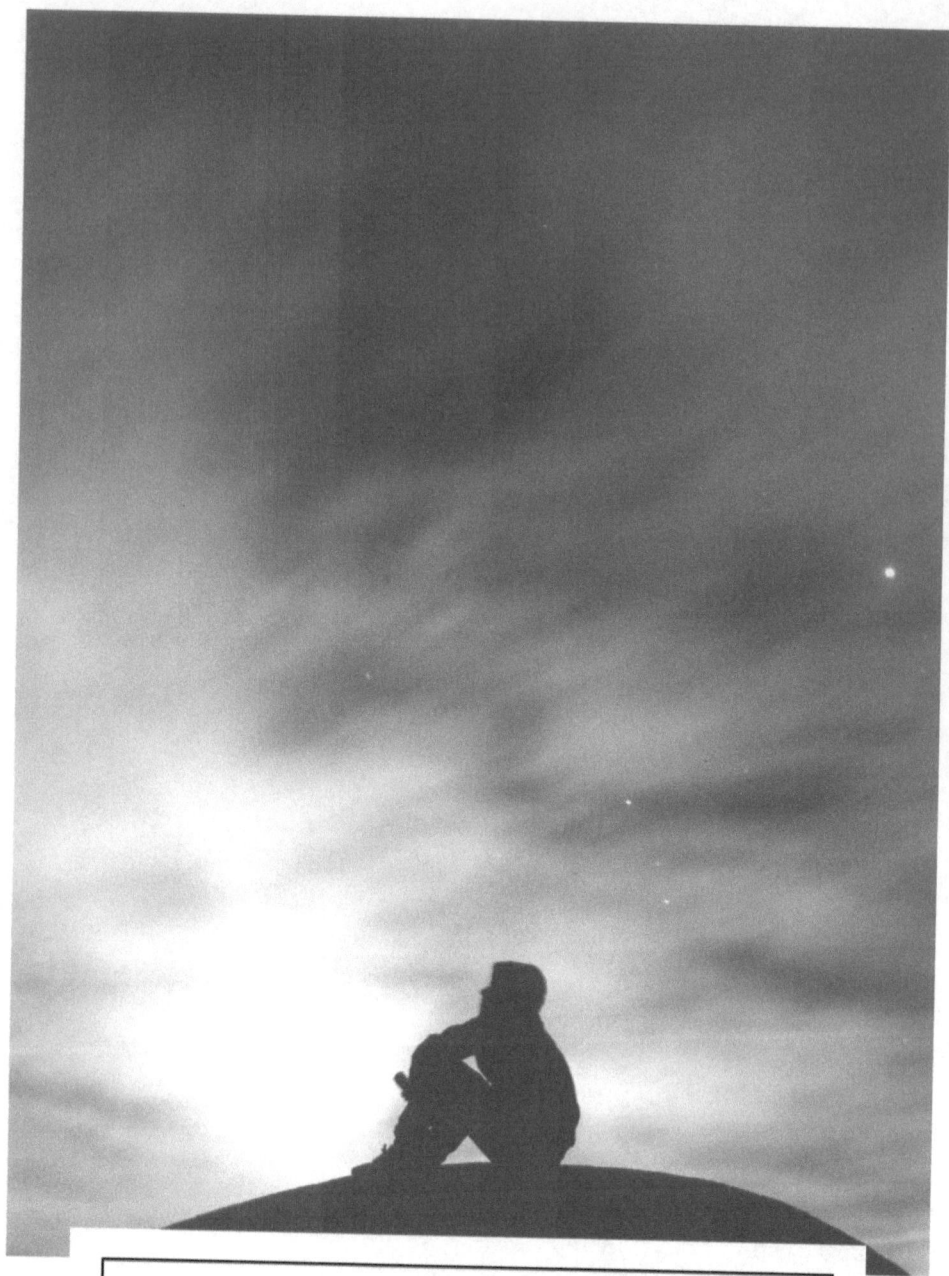

FINAL THOUGHTS

FINAL THOUGHTS

In life there are no coincidences. You reading my book is no coincidence either. We must learn all of the "how to's" of survival. We must apply each lesson learned to be the best version of ourselves that we can be. So much sickness, deep sadness, struggling and dis-ease. We are literally being destroyed from both inside and out. It doesn't have to be this way. We are all better than this. We are all capable of change. Armed now with your survival kit, what will you choose to do? You're not alone. I'm walking out this journey too. Here are some tips to get you started:

- Stay aware
- Get healthy
- Ask questions
- Watch your environment
- Always be prepared
- Stay clean
- Don't take on more than you can handle
- Educate yourself
- Seek to address the root cause of the issue
- Don't fear
- Get rid of the sugar and process foods
- Eat REAL food
- Get rid of distractions
- Be brave and have courage
- Be patient with yourself. Change is a journey.
- Monitor the people you have in your life
- Understand the value of fasting, prayer, and meditation

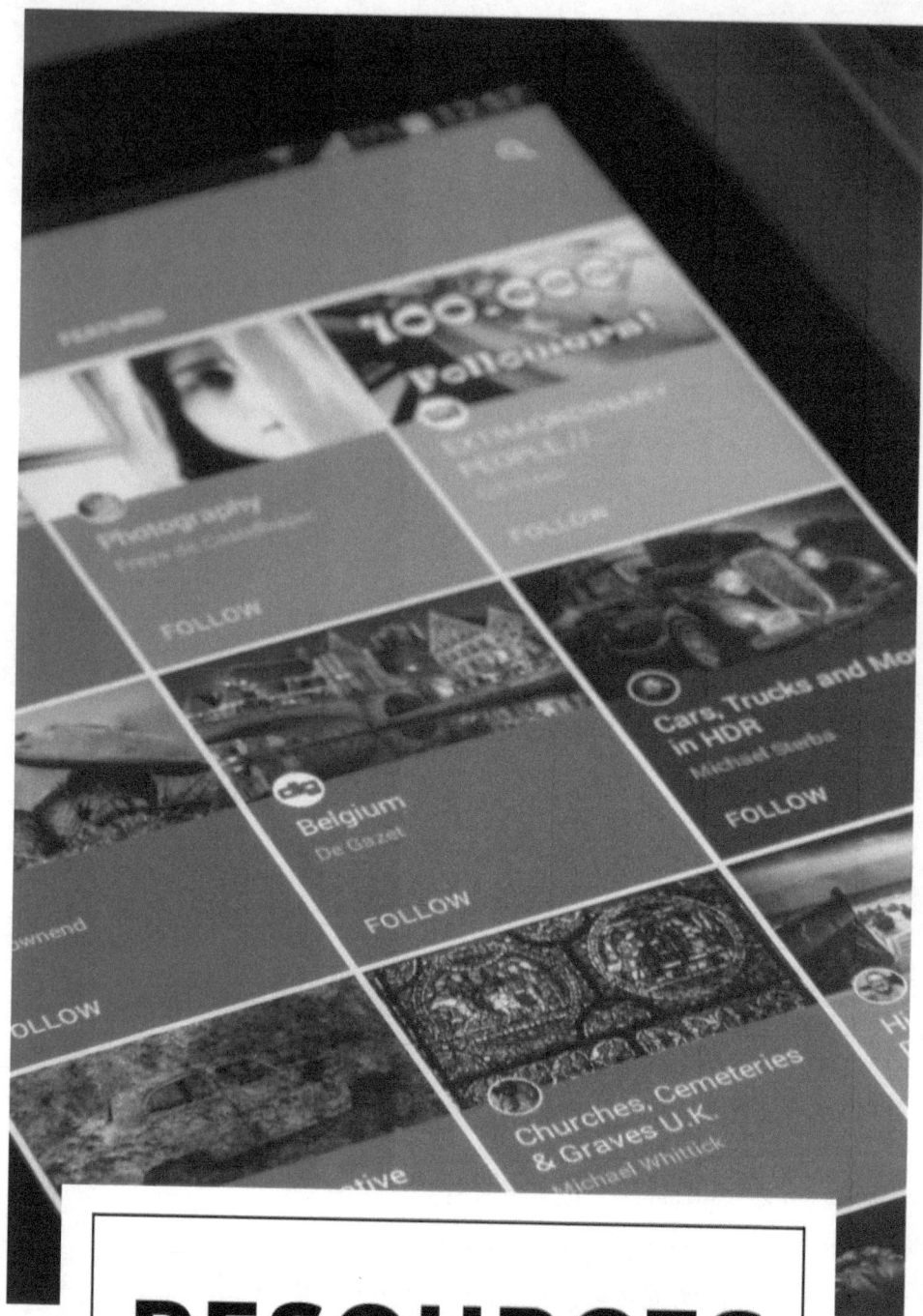

RESOURCES

EMERGENCY NUMBERS

Emergency Medical: 911

Poison control: (800) 222-1222

Animal Poison Control (ASPCA): (888) 426-4435

United States Department of Agriculture(USDA Number): (202) 720-2791

American Red Cross: 1 (800) 733-2767

Coast Guard: VHF-FM Channel 16 (156.8 MHz), dial 911)

Emergency Radio stations: Emergency radio transmission is VHF Channel 16 (156.800 MHz).)

National Weather Service: (815)-834-0675

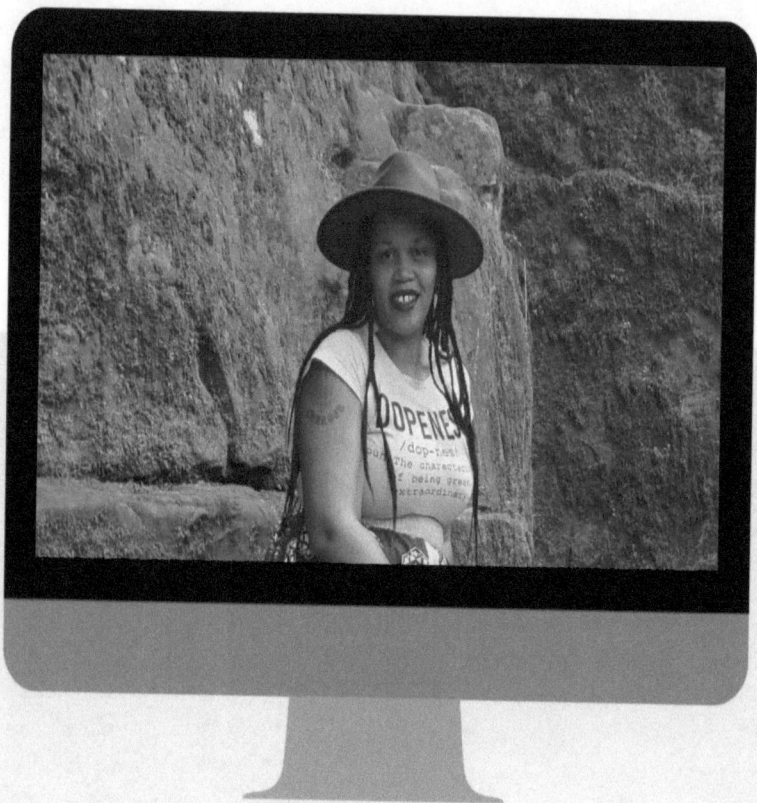

THANK YOU!

This book was created as a labor of love. Thank you for your purchase. I pray this book will guide you through trying times. I look forward to hearing how you discovered a healthier, more confident you!

Enjoy!!!

WWW.THEDEMYSTIFIEDHERBALIST.COM

Glossary

Cardiovascular System- The blood circulatory system (cardiovascular system) that delivers nutrients and oxygen to all cells in the body.

Compress- A cloth soaked in a strong tea and applied on top of your skin.

Creams- Thick substance that consists of water, carrier oils and essential oils.

Decoctions- Herbs placed in water and boiled for a specified time.

Digestive System- Consists of organs that take in food and liquids and break them down into substances that the body can use for energy, growth, and tissue repair.

Douche- A water or cleansing solution designed to go into the vagina of a woman.

Endocrine System- A network of glands and organs that uses hormones to control and coordinate your body's metabolism, energy level, reproduction, growth and development, and response to injury, stress levels, and mood.

Enemas- Injections of fluids used to cleanse or stimulate the emptying of your bowels.

Essential oil- Concentrated aromatic oils distilled from plants.

Excretory System- A system that removes excess and waste products from the body to maintain homeostasis.

First degree burns- Also called a superficial burn, only affects the outer layer of skin.

Foraging- Searching for wild food resources.

Inflammation- A normal part of the body defense to injury or infection.

Infused oil- Plant prepared in a fixed oil (i.e., coconut oil, for external use).

Integumentary System- The skin. It's the largest organ of the body that forms a physical barrier between the external environment and the internal environment that it serves to protect and maintain the body's balance.

Liniment- Plants prepared in isopropyl (rubbing) alcohol (for external use).

Lymphatic System- The tissues and organs that produce, store, and carry white blood cells that fight infections and other diseases.

Medicinal Wines- Soaking herbs in rice, sorghum wine, other alcohol.

Muscular System- Composed of specialized cells called muscle fibers. They are responsible for movement.

Nervous System- Includes the brain, spinal cord, and a complex network of nerves. This system sends messages back and forth between the brain and the body.

Ointments- Steeping herbs in a carrier oil (oil or beeswax).

Parasites- An organism that lives on or in a host organism and gets its food from or at the expense of its host.

Plant based soaps- Plants that have saponins (bubbly stuff that makes soap).

Poison- A substance that is causing the illness of a living organism when introduced or absorbed.

Poultice- Plants cut up and/or cooked and applied topically.

Powder- Plants ground into powder form.

Psychological first aid- An evidence-informed approach that is built on the concept of human resilience in coping with trauma.

Purification tablets- Tablets that contain the disinfectants iodine or chlorine. They can be added to untreated water to kill harmful microorganisms and make the water safer to drink.

Reproductive System- The tissues, glands, and organs involved in producing offspring (children).

Respiratory System- The organs that are involved in breathing. They include the nose, throat, larynx, trachea, bronchi, and lungs. Also called respiratory tract.

Salve- An infused oil with beeswax added.

Second degree burn- This type of burn affects both the epidermis and the second layer of skin (dermis).

Shock- Critical condition brought on by the sudden drop in blood flow through the body.

Skeletal System- Your body's central framework. It consists of bones and connective tissue, including cartilage, tendons, and ligaments.

Soak- A strong tea where the body part is placed directly in the fluid.

Suppositories- A form of medicine contained in a small piece of solid material such as cocoa butter or glycerin and inserted in the rectum.

Syrups- Decocted herbs steeped in sugar or honey.

Tea- Plants prepared in water.

Therapeutic Actions- A word used to describe a specific medicinal property or quality of a plant.

Third degree burn- A third-degree burn destroys your first three layers of skin and fatty tissue.

Tincture- Plants prepared in ethanol (drinking alcohol).

Urinary System- The organs that make urine and remove it from the body.

Washes- Herbs infused in rose water, aloe etc.